VITALITY!

How to Get it and Keep it:
A Homeopath's Guide to
Vibrant Health Without Drugs

VITALITY!
How to Get it and Keep it:
A Homeopath's Guide to
Vibrant Health Without Drugs

Kathleen K. Fry, MD, CTHHom

Collette Avenue Press, LLC
Scottsdale, Arizona

Cover Design by: Rosalyn Migdal and Betsy Kolt
Cover Layout by: Rosalyn Migdal and Betsy Kolt
Cover Photographer: © George Doyle
Author Photograph: © Maggie McDonald - MaggieMcDonald.com
Illustration Credits: © Edward Hamilton

ISBN: 978-0-9847534-0-6

DEDICATION

For Sweet "I are not a" Baby James
and
for Richard, of blessed memory.

TABLE OF CONTENTS

ARE YOU TRULY ALIVE? 1

THE SPIRITUAL VITAL FORCE 9

WHAT IS HOMEOPATHY? 17

CASE STORIES: Real People, Real Problems 31

FREQUENTLY ASKED QUESTIONS 45

HOW DOES HOMEOPATHY DIFFER FROM 47
NATUROPATHY AND HERBAL MEDICINE?

THE HOMEOPATHIC PROCESS 51

WHAT TO EXPECT FROM TREATMENT 55

DO IT YOURSELF EMERGENCY AND 59
ACUTE HOMEOPATHIC CARE

ACUTE REMEDIES FOR CHILDREN 77

ACUTE REMEDIES FOR WOMEN 83

CONCLUSION 93

ARE YOU TRULY ALIVE?

When was the last time you awakened in the morning clear headed, pain free, fully refreshed and energized? Do you jump out of bed ready to take on the world? Or, like so many clients I have seen in my clinic, do you have too many boxes checked on the "My Life Would be Great Except For…" list below?

☐ TIRED ALL THE TIME

☐ CHRONIC PAIN

☐ DEPRESSED

☐ ANXIOUS

☐ PLAGUED BY ALLERGIES

☐ NO SEX DRIVE

☐ CAN'T GET PREGNANT

☐ NEVER WELL SINCE VACCINATION

☐ MENOPAUSAL HORMONE "HELL"

The number of clients I have seen over the years suffering from these ailments and more is well in the tens of thousands. It seems that more often than not, for most people this is their "normal' state of being. On those rare occasions when they do awaken feeling great, they often feel that "it's a fluke" and the next day they go right back to feeling horrible.

What if you could make those rare, wonderful days your new normal and feel great all the time? Imagine what your life would be like if you didn't have to spend so much time in doctors' offices. Think about what else you could do with all of the money you now spend on prescription drugs and inflated health insurance premiums. What would your day be like without having to take a handful of pills each day to "jump start" your heart or your colon? Imagine being clear-headed and happy without having to take psychiatric medications.

Even if you have struggled for years with such "incurable" conditions as Chronic Fatigue Syndrome, Fibromyalgia and Irritable Bowel Syndrome, you do NOT have to suffer any longer. It is possible for you to enjoy a lifetime of good health *without having to swallow a handful of pills several times a day.* I see this happen in my clinic every day and I experience it myself. But it was not always this way.

As a medical student, I found the study of the human body interesting, but it struck me that what we were learning was very mechanical. We started our training by dissecting a cadaver and focusing on learning the names and the functions of all the parts. The thinking is that if we could understand the anatomy and physiology of every cell of the body, then we could learn to fix people when they got sick: sort of like repairing a car or a bicycle. But I had questions that conventional medicine could not answer to my satisfaction.

- What is health?
- Is it more than just the absence of disease?
- Why do we get sick in the first place?
- Why is it that a person's health tends to decline with age?

If this is the natural progression of aging, how do you explain the longevity of certain cultures where people consistently live over 100 years?

It wasn't until I had a class with Dr. Andrew Weil that I realized there were more ways to approach health and healing than just the use of pharmaceutical drugs and surgery. His classes at the University of Arizona College of Medicine were some of the most interesting ones I took in medical school and I recall thinking, "When I get out of here I can do medicine in a different way." But I had no idea about what that would look like and I was still in my training phase.

For most physicians, medical school is just the beginning of their training. Most go on to residency programs to learn a specialty. In allopathic medicine, the focus is on healing the body as if it were a machine.

To do this, physicians are trained to focus on the minutiae of the body and its functions. This detail tends to overwhelm the conscious mind and can lead to feeling overwhelmed by the vast amount of information that needs to be absorbed; hence the specialization of medicine, where the focus is narrowed to a manageable amount of material. Thus, one doctor focuses on the nervous system, another masters the GI tract and still others specialize in surgery.

Within these broad specialties, there are many sub-specialties such as Orthopedics or Pediatric Cardiology. There are even physicians who spend their entire careers focused on the anterior chamber of the eye.

Obstetrics and Gynecology appealed to the generalist in me because, like the Humanities I studied in college, it's a broad specialty that includes medicine, surgery and psychiatry—and you get to deliver babies! I think it's the most joyful of specialties in that most of my clients are genuinely interested in living a healthy lifestyle.

So off I went to the Medical College of Virginia in Richmond to do my specialty training at one of the busiest Ob/Gyn residencies in the country. The sheer volume of patients we saw each day made for a great learning opportunity but the pace was brutal. We were on call in the hospital, up all night caring for very sick patients, every three days. This often meant working 36 hours straight without any sleep. I remember being so tired that I actually fell asleep while dictating an operative note for a Cesarean section I had done in the middle of the night. The hospital transcriptionist called me downstairs the next day to hear myself switch from the details of the operation to dictating my dream.

One benefit of this type of training is that I learned to be a "power-napper'. When I'm tired, I can sleep deeply for 15 or 20 minutes and then I'm good to go for a few more hours.

After I finished my residency, my husband and I moved back to Arizona and I joined a group practice with three other doctors. Though my training had been long and rigorous, I was grateful for it. Even though I was a newly minted doctor, I knew there was nothing in my specialty I would see in Scottsdale that I hadn't already mastered in that giant hospital in Richmond.

To this day, more than twenty-seven years later, I am grateful for all the patients I cared for in those wards and clinics. It was by caring for them that I learned my craft. This knowledge formed the foundation for what has been a very satisfying career.

Despite excellent education and training at some of the finest medical institutions in America, I still felt that something was missing. This became more and more apparent to me as I saw women in my own clinic. Women would come in with various complaints and I would give them medications or perform surgery. Their symptoms would go away for a while. But invariably, after a few months they would be back with a new problem for which I would prescribe more medications.

Oftentimes, they would develop side effects from the medications and then require other drugs to treat the side effects. Increasingly it felt as if I were playing a losing game of "Whack-a Mole", the carnival game where you keep hitting creatures with a mallet. Each time you whack one down, another pops up. I often felt that conventional medicine was a similar game. Symptoms kept popping up no matter what I prescribed.

I saw people developing more symptoms, seeing more specialists and taking more medications. Some of my older clients were taking as many as fifteen different medications a day. I thought to myself, "There has to be a better way" and I remembered the promise I had made to myself as a medical student to find a way to care for people that made sense to me.

I still had not found the answers to the questions I had in medical school. How can it be that two children with the same parents, growing up in the same home and eating the same food, could have completely different states of health? While one daughter was healthy and athletic, her sister was sickly with low energy, terrible menstrual cramps and chronic headaches. It had to be something more than just genetics and environment.

So I began to read. One of the first books that helped me re-examine my approach to health and healing was *Love, Medicine and Miracles* by Dr. Bernie Siegel. Dr. Siegel is a brilliant surgeon who, at the time, specialized in the surgical treatment of cancer at Yale Medical School. My cousin, an oncology nurse, recommended that I read it.

Early in the book, Bernie talks about the client who approached him in the store and asked, "Hey, Doc, remember me? Thirteen years ago you told me that I had six months to live!" That was the beginning of Bernie's search for the true nature of healing, and Bernie's book was the beginning for me.

The book jacket said that in addition to his work at Yale, Bernie was co-president with Dr. Christianne Northrup of the American Holistic Medical Association (AHMA). I had never heard of this organization but wanted to learn more. I phoned Bernie's office at Yale and was referred to the AHMA headquarters in Seattle. The kind woman on the phone explained to me that the AHMA is a national organization of MDs and DOs who are interested in treating the whole person: body, mind and spirit.

It was news to me that there was a group of physicians committed to such a concept and I was immediately intrigued. Perhaps this is where I would find the answers to my questions? So I registered for their upcoming annual meeting that happened to be in Seattle in February. Growing up in California and Arizona, I had never been to Seattle, much less in the middle of winter. I didn't see the sun once the entire week I was there. But it was one of the best weeks I ever spent anywhere.

For the first time since college, I found like-minded people who had the same questions and doubts about conventional medicine as I did. That first week, I did a Vision Quest with a shaman, learned about Healing Touch and participated in a "Healing with Humor" workshop with Patch Adams who was dressed in full clown regalia. Clearly, this was *not* your conventional medical conference.

I felt that I had come home. I later served on the AHMA Board of Trustees for thirteen years, eventually being elected to serve a three-year term as President. I flew all over the country for board meetings three times a year and made some lifelong friendships. Through yearly conferences and workshops with holistic physicians from all over the world, I received what amounted to a second medical education akin to that undertaken by naturopaths. I learned about nutrition and how to assess clients for nutritional deficiencies.

I learned how to evaluate people for food allergies, leaky gut syndrome, and lactose intolerance. I learned the safe and effective way to treat symptoms of menopause using Bio-Identical Hormone therapy from Dr. Jonathan Wright who pioneered the technique. I became familiar with new laboratories that offered more comprehensive testing for conditions that I had never learned in conventional medical school. I was approached by a major nutritional supplement company from Japan and asked to design a formula that would help women with the symptoms of menopause.

With the help of Claudia Wingo, R.N., a nurse and master herbalist we formulated a product called "Estrologic" that has helped thousands of women to make a smooth transition through menopause.

Yet, I still wasn't satisfied. Yes, I was able to help people in ways that I had not been able to help them before but I still felt that something was missing. True, I was prescribing fewer medications for my clients, but now I was loading them up with herbs and supplements.

I felt that my approach, while broader than previously, was still more like a shotgun than a laser beam. I had a better idea of how a healthy human body functions, but I was still not any closer to understanding the *mystery* of how we heal.

As I usually do when I need guidance, I turned to prayer and just before I went to the annual AHMA meeting in 1989, I asked God to show me a system of healing that I could use that was consistent and that I could learn. My prayer went something like this: "Dear God, Creator of the Universe, if you were a sick human being, what system would YOU use to heal yourself?" I promised to keep my eyes and ears open as I went back to Seattle, once again in dreary February.

I don't believe in coincidence. I found myself "by mistake" in a workshop about Homeopathy because the workshop for which I had originally registered was cancelled when the instructor got snowed-in in Minnesota. So it was a prayer and a blizzard that led me to my first lecture on Homeopathy.

As Dr. Linda Johnston, a medical doctor and homeopath, from Los Angeles explained the history and principles of Homeopathy, a feeling in my gut said, "This is it. The answer to my prayer."

I became a student of Homeopathy and initially studied with several teachers until I met Vega Rozenberg and became a student at ESSH, Evolution of the Self School of Homeopathy. Homeopathy is the most powerful form of healing that I have ever encountered. I finally have the answers to the questions I had as a first year medical student.

I have been able to help people in ways that I never could with conventional medicine. I no longer perform surgery, even though I am a skilled surgeon and I enjoyed it, because I have come to understand that removing healthy organs is not only detrimental to a person's overall health, it is largely unnecessary except in extreme cases. When properly applied in a timely fashion, Homeopathy restores a being to health without the suppressive effects of drugs or surgery.

In 1997, I became severely fatigued as a result of overwork in a very stressful environment. Despite feeling exhausted I could barely sleep. I knew that Homeopathy could help me and so I consulted Vega Rozenberg, the Chancellor of ESSH. Several people whom I trusted recommended him. Vega took my case and recommended a remedy for me, which I began taking immediately and slept like a baby for the first time in months, awakening refreshed. I am deeply grateful for what Homeopathy and Vega have and continued to do for me. I have not taken a prescription drug in over twenty years and I enjoy vibrant good health. This excellent state of health and vitality is what I wish for all people and it is possible for all of us to have it.

THE SPIRITUAL VITAL FORCE

Not only is this state of vibrant emotional and physical health possible, it is also absolutely necessary in order for you to fulfill your soul's true purpose.

We are spirit beings inhabiting "skin suits," our bodies. The body does not run itself. It is controlled by an unseen power that Samuel Hahnemann, the father of Homeopathy, termed the "Vital Force": the "spirit-like *dynamis* that rules the body with unbounded sway." It is the force that traditional Chinese physicians call *chi* and the Ayurvedic physicians of India call *prana*.

What does this mean in our daily lives? Every second of every minute of every hour of every day, our bodies perform many, many functions without our conscious control. Imagine if you consciously had to make bone marrow, digest breakfast, remodel your colon, and grow hair and toe nails—you would have no time to use a computer, read a book, compose a symphony, or even just take out the trash.

All of the wondrous things that our bodies do without our conscious input are under the control of the Vital Force. But unlike functions of the body that can be measured with blood tests, evaluated with CT scans, or examined by doctors, the Vital Force is *unseen*. It is only by observing its *effects* that we are able to assess its strength.

You can feel when your own Vital Force is strong and when it is weak. When it is strong, you awaken refreshed after a night of deep, satisfying sleep. You get out of bed easily, without pain in your back or your joints, and you can start your day *without needing any pills*. When the Vital Force is strong and healthy, you don't have to take medications or other substances to "crank up" your colon or to wake up. *You are already* awake, alive, and ready to go.

When you have a strong Vital Force, you feel balanced

emotionally and have a reservoir of patience that allows you to be kind and loving with your family members, friends, colleagues, and even casual acquaintances. You've probably experienced just the opposite condition at times in your life.

When the Vital Force is weak and unhealthy, you can't sleep well. You toss and turn or wake up in the middle of the night and can't go back to sleep unless you take a pill—and even that doesn't always work. When you lack essential vitality, you have stiff joints or aching muscles and wish you could just stay in bed. You feel cranky, irritable, and sometimes quite *angry* about how you feel. So your family members walk around "on eggshells," because they've learned that if they cross you, there will be hell to pay.

When you feel this exhausted, your sex drive is gone. Without vitality, you don't have the emotional stamina to support those who rely on you for strength: your family, your friends and your coworkers.

Without a well functioning Vital Force, you cannot fulfill your soul's purpose. What does this mean? It means that each of us is born as the Bible says, in the image of the Creator. As one of my teachers, Vega Rozenberg has explained it on numerous occasions at his homeopathic school ESSH, "You are born to create and to re-create." You are born to fulfill your soul's destiny. Your task as a human is to learn what that destiny is and to attain it. You have been given certain skills and talents, and if you pay attention to and follow the guidance of your heart, you will discover what it is that you were born to do.

Michael Jordan was not born to be a North Carolina fireman, or a world famous chef, and certainly not a curveball-hitting outfielder for the Chicago White Sox. By following his passion for basketball, he developed his innate talents to become the greatest athlete of his time. And that required *vitality* in addition to vision, drive, and commitment. If, God forbid, he had been born sickly, or his parents had failed to feed him properly, we would never have known his name.

It is not enough to be born with talent. That talent needs to be discovered, nurtured, and developed. And when that happens, mastery and magic occur. You have your own set of innate abilities, the mastery of which contributes to the betterment of the world. You don't have to be a Michael Jordan to make a big difference in your own life and the lives of those you love. But you *must* have the vitality and stamina to do what you need to do.

The Vital Force or Spirit follows certain Universal Laws or Principles. Although we cannot see, touch, taste, or smell them, we can and do observe the effects of these Principles on our lives each day. The Vital Force governs every cell of our beings. It is that unseen Force that tells our cells to divide in two instead of three, or four, or seven. It is what guides the sperm to find the egg and begin the process of creating an entire human being "from scratch". It is what gives us the patience to read "Goodnight, Moon" to our toddlers over and over again, night after night after night.

Like the body, the Vital Force requires care and feeding. Certain things build the Vital Force, and other things drain it. Let's look first at those things that diminish the Vital Force— what I call *vitality suckers.*

VITALITY SUCKERS

Vitality suckers generally are toxic, such as alcohol and illegal drugs. But it also includes things we don't normally think of as toxic, such as pharmaceutical drugs. The latter, *designed to suppress symptoms*, ultimately deplete the Vital Force.

All pharmaceutical drugs are suppressive, removing symptoms by driving spiritual disease responsible for the symptoms deeper into the body. For example, a urinary tract infection might occur when the Vital Force is weak, leading to a weakening of the immune system, which, in its healthy state, removes bacteria that don't belong in the bladder or kidneys.

Antibiotic drugs override the immune system and attack the bacteria but do nothing to strengthen the Vital Force responsible for maintaining the immune system in optimal working order. But a properly chosen homeopathic remedy stimulates the Vital Force, which will mobilize the immune system.

Rather than overriding the immune system and killing the bacteria, as do antibiotics, homeopathic remedies strengthen the

Vital Force. The result is an optimally functioning immune system that produces many white blood cells to destroy the bacteria, restoring the urine to its normal sterile state and preventing recurring infections.

Pharmaceutical drugs weaken the Vital Force because they are foreign substances that override the workings of the Spiritual Vital Force. The Vital Force is like the conductor of a symphony, directing *in concert* all of the necessary functions of the physical body. When the Vital Force is strong and healthy, it directs each cell of the body to perform its functions in vibrant harmony with all of the other cells of the body.

There are many other vitality suckers, such as a spouse who belittles you by calling you "stupid" or one who is so busy looking after the kids that there's no time or attention left for you. Or a boss who is under so much pressure to perform that he drives you right to the brink. Or a coworker who gossips about everyone in the office and leaves you feeling demoralized just from listening.

Eating unhealthy food, not getting enough fresh air and exercise, working too much, and worrying about all sorts of things are among the many things people can do to themselves that deplete their vitality.

In my capacity as a physician and homeopath, working mostly with women, each day I see the effects of depleted vitality.

Here are two of the most common "syndromes" I see virtually every day; do you recognize yourself?

OVER-EXERCISERS

Prior to my recent move to Boulder, Colorado I worked for twenty-seven years in Scottsdale, Arizona where the weather is usually wonderful, attracting people from all over the world who come to hike in the Grand Canyon, raft down the Colorado River, and climb beautiful mountains. In moderation, these are all good things. But like so many good things, they can be taken to extremes. And when they are, the ill effects would show up in my office.

I recently saw a woman who is physically in great condition

but looks about a dozen years older than her actual age. She taught aerobics and spin classes for more than two decades, and she came to see me mainly because of exhaustion and horrible symptoms during the approach of menopause.

She was taking Advil for chronic joint pain. Her diet was awful—she never ate breakfast and lived mainly on energy drinks and candy. Like many over-exercisers, she struggled with various eating disorders. She has hot flashes all day, and night sweats disrupt her sleep throughout the night. She's extremely irritable, especially during the week before her menses. And despite years of heavy exercise, she actually has bone loss.

I notice this a lot at my health club, and maybe you've noticed it at yours: those who are first on the treadmill at 5:30 every morning or take two spin classes a day all look older than they are, and their skin tends to be wrinkled and lacks a healthy color. Like my aerobics-teaching client, they are addicted to their own adrenaline. Over the years they have depleted their Spiritual Vital Force by over taxing their bodies.

SELF-MEDICATORS

When people lack vitality, they develop symptoms. These symptoms can be physical, mental, or emotional. We all try to make ourselves feel better when we don't feel well, and this leads to self-medication. People medicate themselves with a wide variety of things. Some people overeat. Others try drugs, either illegal or pharmaceutical, which temporarily suppress symptoms. As detailed above, *all* drugs do *nothing* to relieve the *cause* of the symptoms. In fact, over time they lead to ill health because they deplete the Spiritual Vital Force.

This is very commonly the case for patients who take numerous medications. Consider the people you know who go to doctors frequently. Are they the healthiest people you know? Most likely, they are not. If health and vitality came in pills, then the healthiest people would be those taking the most medications, yet we know that is not the case.

Some people "medicate" their symptoms not with drugs, but with shopping, going into debt for a closet full of shoes or to own $1,000.00 handbags when they already have dozens. Other people treat their symptoms with sex or pornography. This can lead to problems with relationships, sexually transmitted infections, and even legal troubles. Why do people engage in such behaviors? The bottom line is that *their Vital Force is weak*—like an out of tune orchestra, there is chaos instead of harmony.

Over-medicators are desperately trying to restore their inner harmony. But their behaviors don't accomplish that, because *they don't affect* the source of the problem. They do nothing to strengthen the Vital Force. During more than twenty-seven years as a physician, I have seen thousands of women in varying stages of depletion and exhaustion. It is especially apparent when women approach the menopause that the true state of the Vital Force is revealed.

So, if allopathic, conventional medicine merely suppresses symptoms, what can we use to restore ourselves to health and maintain our vitality? After many years of searching I discovered the answer and have used it exclusively for myself and my family for more than twenty years: Homeopathy.

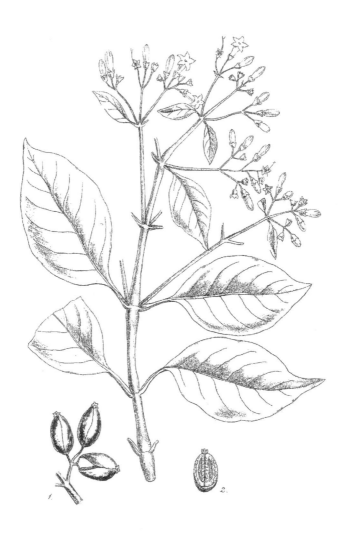

CHINA OFFICINALIS

WHAT IS HOMEOPATHY?

Homeopathy is a form of healing that uses natural substances prepared in a special way in a homeopathic pharmacy, to strengthen the SPIRITUAL Vital Force and restore us to health.

Homeopathy comes from the Greek words "homeos", meaning "similar," and "pathos", meaning "suffering." Homeopathy works on the principle that *like heals like*: a substance that brings on a set of symptoms when given to a healthy person can be used to strengthen the Vital Force in a person exhibiting those same symptoms. As the Spiritual Vital Force is restored, the symptoms diminish and eventually disappear.

The power of homeopathic remedies is revealed when volunteers take them in a process known as a *proving*. The information gathered in the proving of a large number of natural substances is recorded in what is known as the *Materia Medica*. This body of knowledge allows a homeopath to choose from more than 5,000 remedies in order to annihilate disease and restore vibrant health, as described in this book.

THE HISTORY OF HOMEOPATHY

How did Homeopathy come about? This is one of the most fascinating, yet widely unknown stories in the history of Western medicine. Samuel Hahnemann (b.1755–d.1843) was a physician who lived and worked in Germany, primarily in Saxony. He was appalled by the techniques that passed for healing treatment by the doctors of his time. In those days, disease was thought to be due to an imbalance of the four "humors": black bile (melan chole), yellow bile (chole), phlegm (phlegma) and blood (sanguis). This theory had been the basis of medical practice since the time of Hippocrates.

Treatments were designed to restore the balance of these humors by such drastic means as sweating, purging, vomiting, and bloodletting. Toxic substances such as arsenic and mercury were used to treat diseases such as syphilis, which was rampant throughout Europe in the 18th century.

Hahnemann saw that the treatments were often worse than the diseases they were attempting to eliminate. So he quit the practice of medicine. But he had a wife and seven children to feed, so he supported his family by translating into German ancient medical texts written in Greek and Latin by such luminaries as Hippocrates, Galen, and Paracelsus.

During this time of intensive study, Hahnemann realized a deep truth that would lead to a radical new system of healing.

In the Introduction to the *Organon of Medicine, 6th Edition,* Hahnemann explains: "As long as men have existed they have been liable, individually or collectively to diseases from physical or moral causes. In a rude state of nature but few remedial agents were required, as the simple mode of living admitted of but few disease; with the civilization of mankind in the state, on the contrary, the occasions of diseases and the necessity for medical aid increased in equal proportion. But ever since that time (soon after Hippocrates, therefore, for 2500 years) men have occupied themselves with the treatment of ever increasing multiplicity of diseases, who led astray by their vanity, sought by reasoning and guessing to excogitate the mode of furnishing this aid. *Innumerable and dissimilar ideas* respecting the nature of diseases and their remedies sprang from so many dissimilar brains, and the theoretical views these gave rise to the so-called systems, each of which was at variance with the rest and self-contradictory." (Italics added.)

This continued to be true in Hahnemann's time when there was no innate understanding of how the body healed or what caused people to be sick. New treatments were being introduced arbitrarily based on nothing but conjecture and speculation.

An unexpected development occurred about the same time that led Hahnemann to create an entirely new system of healing and to return him to caring for patients. In 1790, Hahnemann was translating the *Materia Medica* of William Cullen, a Scottish physician, from English into German. Cullen maintained that Peruvian Cinchona (quinine) bark was effective for treating malaria because of its tonic effect on the stomach. Hahnemann was unconvinced of this because there were many so-called "stomach tonics" that were not effective in treating malaria.

He decided to experiment on himself and proceeded to take small amounts of quinine bark for several days. What do you suppose happened? If you guessed that he developed the symptoms of malaria, you would be right. Mind you, the malarial parasite wasn't identified until nearly a century later.

In Hahnemann's time, no one knew about the association between malaria and mosquitoes. Without being bitten by a parasite-carrying mosquito, Hahnemann developed a full-blown case of malaria, with its distinctly characteristic fever alternating with chills and delirium. How could this happen? By taking this substance, Hahnemann was able to discover the innate healing power of the quinine bark.

This extraordinary development was actually the first proving of a homeopathic remedy. Hahnemann kept meticulous notes about his symptoms, including the subjects of his dreams, the foods he craved, his moods, and his thinking patterns.

This record became the first entry in the Homeopathic *Materia Medica*, and the remedy is known today as CHINA OFFICINALIS. Not only does it successfully restore the Vital Force of a person with symptoms of malaria, it is also a very effective remedy for weakness brought on by loss of bodily fluids. It is one of our most important remedies for postpartum hemorrhage and subsequent anemia.

Once Hahnemann discovered the power of the proving process, he began to test other substances, including the most commonly prescribed medicines of his day, including arsenic and mercury. Hahnemann cataloged the underlying principles of Homeopathy in a book called the *Organon of Medicine*. In the very first paragraph of this work, Hahnemann clearly stated the *raison d'être* for every physician: *"The physician's high and only mission is to restore the sick to health, to cure, as it is termed."*

Notice that Hahnemann did *not* say: "The physician's high and only mission is to keep people on many medications for their entire lives, with continued decline in their health." In fact, Hahnemann said just the *opposite* (*Organon, 6th Edition*, paragraph 9):

"In the healthy condition of man, the spiritual vital force (autocracy), the dynamis that animates the material body (organism) rules with unbounded sway, and retains all the parts of the organism in admirable, harmonious, vital operation, as regards both sensations and functions, *so that* our indwelling, reason-gifted mind can freely employ this living, healthy instrument for the higher purposes of our *existence*."

Hahnemann explained the fallacy of conventional medicine in the *Organon, 6th Edition,* (paragraph 23):

"All pure experience, however, and all accurate research convince us that persistent symptoms of disease are far from being removed and annihilated by *opposite* symptoms of medicines (as in the *antipathic, enantiopathic,* or *palliative* method), that, on the contrary, after transient, apparent alleviation, they break forth again, only with increased intensity and become manifestly aggravated." ('Antipathic' is what we today call allopathic, or conventional, medicine.)

HOW DO WE KNOW WHICH REMEDIES TO USE?

How is it that we know what the Vital Force needs? How do we know which remedies can be used to completely annihilate disease and restore people to health? By testing natural substances on healthy people, as Hahnemann discussed in paragraph 107 of the *Organon, 6th Edition*:

"If, in order to ascertain [the pathogenetic effects of medicines to be used for healing], medicines be given to *sick* persons, only, even though they be administered singly, and alone, then little or nothing precise is seen of their true effects, as those peculiar alterations of the health to be expected from the medicine are mixed up with the symptoms of the disease and can seldom be distinctly observed."

And in paragraph 108:

"There is, therefore, no other possible way in which the peculiar effects of medicines on the health of individuals can be accurately ascertained—there is no sure, no more natural way of accomplishing this object, than to administer the several medicines experimentally, in moderate doses, to *healthy* persons, in order to ascertain what changes, symptoms, and signs of their influence each individually produces on the health of the body and of the mind; that is to say, what disease elements they are able and tend to produce, since, as has been demonstrated [in Paragraphs 24-27], all the curative power of medicines lies in this power they possess of changing the state of man's health, and it is revealed by observation of the latter".

Paragraph 20:

"This spirit-like power to alter man's state of health which lies hidden in the inner nature of medicines can in itself never be discovered by us by a mere effort of reason; it is only by experience of the phenomena *it displays* when acting on the state of health of man that we can become clearly cognizant of it."

Paragraph 21:

"…so it follows that when medicines act as remedies, they can only bring their curative property into play by means of this their power of altering man's state of health by the production of peculiar symptoms; and that, therefore, we have only to rely on the morbid phenomena which the medicines produce in the healthy body as the sole possible revelation of their in-dwelling curative power, in order to learn what disease-producing power, and at the same time what disease-curing power, each individual medicine possesses."

Thus, the information obtained during a proving is the only reliable information we can use to know which remedy will act on the Vital Force to restore a person to a state of health by annihilating disease.

HOW IS A PROVING DONE?

The best provings are done over a period of time with healthy volunteers. I'm always suspicious about what I call "drive-by" provings done at weekend conferences.

I'm wary about giving remedies based on information from such provings. The best provings are done by large groups of individuals over periods of time sufficient to observe the effects of the remedy on the mental, emotional and physical aspects of the provers.

HOW IS A PROVING ORGANIZED AND PERFORMED?

Healthy volunteers begin by writing summaries of their current states of health, being sure to record any physical or emotional symptoms they are having prior to the starting of the proving, if any. The volunteers take the remedy being proved, but they have no knowledge of the original substance used to prepare this remedy. The potency given can vary, but the idea is to give a strong enough potency for long enough to produce symptoms in healthy people.

For example, in the proving of ANDROCTONOS, done by Jeremy Sherr and the Dynamis School of Homeopathy, a remedy based on material from a scorpion, twenty-seven volunteers, both male and female, ranging in age from 25 to 40, took the remedy until it produced symptoms.

Three provers took milk sugar as a placebo. Most of the provers took the remedy for 30 days, but some required only six days before symptoms arose. Once symptoms begin to appear, the prover stops taking the remedy.

Each prover keeps very detailed records of everything that happens to him or her during the course of the proving, which could last for several weeks; some symptoms have been known to persist for months. The provers are not allowed to discuss their symptoms with other provers, in order to maintain objective records of their experiences. At the end of the proving, the supervisor collects all of the provers' records and reviews them. The common symptoms reported for each remedy are the basis for the *Materia Medica*.

For example, in the proving of ANDROCTONOS, many of the provers reported a feeling of detachment, depression, or despondency. Many noted that they felt entirely alone in the world—an interesting symptom if you consider that most scorpions travel alone and are rarely seen in packs. Many also reported feelings of irritability and apathy toward the things they usually enjoyed.

Others had dreams of destruction, and one prover had a nightmare in which she dreamed that she had killed her grandfather by poking him in the eye with a knitting needle while he slept. Many provers noted that they had mood swings and were clumsy and accident-prone.

On the other hand, one prover had felt that she could forgive her parents for any real or imagined slights, and "at the same time she felt as though knots were untying within her." So in her case, the remedy was actually beneficial. This is not uncommon in provings, where many instances have been reported of chronic symptoms permanently alleviated.

Hahnemann himself recommended that physicians do provings, and he was responsible for proving more than 100 remedies, mostly on himself, his family, and his students and colleagues. Perhaps this is why he lived to the ripe old age of eighty-eight, a rare feat in the late 18th century, when most men died in their early forties.

There is another way of adding information about remedies to the *Materia Medica* and that is through poisonings or through clinical cures. One of the most famous of these provings was Constantine Hering's accidental proving of LACHESIS. While gathering venom from the Suruku snake, one of the deadliest snakes in South America, Hering was bitten by the snake he was handling. He had a violent reaction, including marked paralysis of the left side of the body.

In fact, almost all his symptoms were on the left side. His wife kept meticulous notes as she observed what must have been a horrible sight. Interestingly, when the Suruku snake swallows a large prey, it disarticulates its jaw, beginning on the left side.

Additional symptoms of some remedies have been added to the *Materia Medica* over the years as homeopaths have observed patients cured of chronic illnesses after taking particular remedies. Despite this helpful information, the gold standard is the proving, as originally delineated by Hahnemann.

HOW ARE REMEDIES MADE?

I'm often asked by clients who are new to Homeopathy, "What's in this remedy pellet?" The simplest, yet most confusing, answer is "Nothing!" Unlike conventional, allopathic medications that contain chemical substances that you can measure in a laboratory, a chemical analysis of a homeopathic remedy will reveal nothing but sugar, water, and alcohol for every remedy. In fact, the chemical signature of every remedy above the 12C potency (see below) would be the same. How can this be? To answer this question, I must explain how remedies are made.

The first step in the production of a remedy is to make a *Mother Tincture*. Mother Tinctures can be made from any substance, including plants, animals, and minerals. (Remedies have even been made from sunlight and from ocean water.)

A Mother Tincture is made by first grinding a substance into a fine powder in a process known as *trituration.* A small amount of the powder is then dissolved in either water or alcohol. For example, in the case of a remedy called AURUM, the Mother Tincture is made by dissolving small grains of pure gold metal in alcohol.

Once the Mother Tincture is made, the homeopathic pharmacist proceeds to make the remedy from the Mother Tincture in the following manner: One drop of the Mother Tincture is added to 99 drops of water, and then the container of liquid is rapped sharply on a surface in a process known as *succession* (Hahnemann was said to have used his family Bible as a succession surface).

This first dilution is labeled "1C" (or sometimes "1Ch"). The "C" stands for centesimal, denoting that each potency has been diluted in 100 drops of water. This distinguishes the potency from a "1X" dilution, which is made using dilutions of 10 drops of water. Then one drop is taken from the 1C dilution, added to 99 drops of water, and succussed; this is a 2C dilution. Successive drops are diluted in 99 drops of water and succussed until the desired dilution is achieved.

The final dilution is then poured onto milk sugar (lactose) pellets or tablets. The pellets are just carriers for the spiritual essence released from the substance during its preparation. One pellet constitutes one dose. How can it be that something so dilute will actually work? As Hahnemann described in his *Organon of Medicine, 6th Edition*, paragraph 269:

"This remarkable change in the qualities of the natural bodies develops the latent, hitherto unperceived, as if slumbering hidden, dynamic powers which influence *THE LIFE PRINCIPLE*, change the well-being of animal life."

Serially diluting and succussing a natural substance releases the healing power of that substance which then stimulates the dynamic, spiritual Vital Force that is responsible for maintaining every being in a state of balanced equipoise.

HOW DO WE KNOW HOMEOPATHY WORKS?

If there is no measurable material substance contained in a remedy, how do we know that a remedy is working? By observing the effects on the person who takes the remedy. Let's look at an example.

Emily is the first-born child and is doted on by her parents, grandparents, aunts, and uncles. For about two years, she is the center of her family's devotion. Then Emily's mother brings home a baby brother, and Emily is no longer the center of everyone's undivided attention. She begins acting out, and mom catches her trying to hurt the baby.

Emily also develops a red, itching rash in patches all over her body. So mom takes her to a pediatrician, who looks at the rash and says, "This is eczema." He prescribes a steroid cream that mom puts on the rash, and it goes away. However, whenever Emily gets upset or overtired, the rash comes back. So mom continues to apply the cream every time the rash comes back, and it temporarily goes away. Fast forward a few years. Emily develops asthma. She goes back to the pediatrician, who now prescribes a steroid inhaler and strong asthma medications to stop the wheezing. Sometimes she requires special breathing treatments. Meanwhile, the rash continues to get worse.

A few years later, Emily goes to school, and her teachers

notice she can't sit still for very long and tends to be irritable and easily upset. A visit to the pediatrician brings a new diagnosis (ADHD—attention deficit hyperactivity disorder) and a new prescription for yet another medication.

When Emily turns twelve, she starts her menses and has horrible cramps, heavy bleeding, and nausea. So her pediatrician prescribes birth control pills to stop the symptoms. Now we have a twelve-year-old child on a cream to suppress the rash, steroids and an inhaler to stop the wheezing, psychiatric medicines to manage her concentration, and birth control pills to suppress her hormonal system and relieve her monthly menstrual pain.

This is a pretty typical scenario for conventional medical practice. Over the course of a lifetime, people like Emily will be on *hundreds* of prescriptions for everything from colds, flu, and ear infections to arthritis and diabetes.

When she reaches seventy, she will most likely be on enough prescriptions that she needs a pill container to keep track of them all. But is she healthy? The answer is *no.* Hahnemann noted similar phenomena 400 years ago, and he described them quite poetically in paragraph 13 of his *Organon*:

"Therefore disease (that does not come within the province of manual surgery) considered, as it is by the allopathists, as a thing separate from the living whole, from the organism and its annihilating vital force, and hidden in the interior, be it of ever so subtle a character, is *an absurdity*, that could only be imagined by minds of a materialistic stamp, and has for *thousands* of years given to the prevailing system of medicine all those *pernicious* impulses that have made it a truly mischievous (non-healing) art."

Remember that in Hahnemann's day the "prevailing system of medicine" included such "pernicious impulses" as bloodletting and purging with mercury and arsenic. We now look in horror at such barbaric treatments, but ask yourself this: "How will the people of the future view the chemotherapy and radiation that we herald today as state of the art in our own "prevailing system of medicine"?

Hahnemann distilled the essence of Homeopathy into one rather meandering paragraph (16 in the 6th Edition of the *Organon*):

"Our vital force, as a spirit-like dynamis, cannot be attacked and affected by injurious influences on the healthy organism caused by the external inimical forces that disturb the harmonious play of life, otherwise than in a *spirit-like* (dynamic) way, and in like manner, all such morbid derangements (diseases) cannot be removed from it by the physician in any other way than by the spirit-like (dynamic virtual) alterative powers of the serviceable medicines (remedies) acting upon our spirit-like vital force, which perceives them through the medium of the sentient faculty of the nerves everywhere present in the organism, so that *it is only by their dynamic action on the vital force* that remedies are to *re-establish* and do actually re-establish health and vital harmony, after the changes in the health of the patient cognizable by our senses (the totality of symptoms) have revealed the disease to the carefully observing and investigating physician as fully as was requisite in order to enable him to cure it."

Essentially, this means that all disease cannot be completely annihilated and the diseased person restored to health, *except* by something that acts on the spirit, or the Vital Force. Thus, remedies must be prepared in such a way that they are able to interact with this spiritual Vital Force. And the only way to know if they are interacting properly with this Vital Force is to observe closely the complete *annihilation* of disease.

This is in complete contrast to allopathic medicine that uses creams to suppress rashes, steroid inhalers to suppress the symptoms of asthma, and anti-depressants and anti-anxiety medicines to suppress mental symptoms. If these drugs were successful in annihilating disease, then when the medications were discontinued, none of the symptoms would return.

But we know from clinical experience that whenever anti-depressants are discontinued, most of the time, the symptoms of depression return, sometimes worse than before. This can doom people to a lifetime of drug taking—and who knows what 30 or 40 years of anti-depressant drugs do to the brain? But almost 400 years ago, Hahnemann had a greater vision of what constituted true healing.

Paragraph 17:

"But when the disease is annihilated, health is restored, and this is the *highest*, sole aim of the physician who knows the true object of his mission, which consists *not in learned-sounding pratting*, but in giving aid to the sick."

How would a homeopath approach Emily's case? The most important information to a homeopath comes by asking the question: What happened to Emily's Spiritual Vital Force when she developed a rash? A good homeopath understands that the rash is a symptom from the Vital Force communicating that something is out of balance in Emily. What is it that caused Emily to develop the rash in the first place?

The birth of Emily's baby brother caused an emotional shift in Emily because she was no longer the sole focus of her family's affections. She really experienced a form of grief over the loss of her exalted position in the family. Her Vital Force communicated that grief by creating a rash.

Notice that the Vital Force didn't give her a brain tumor or a heart attack, just a rash. The reason for this, as observed time and again by working homeopaths, is that *the Vital Force always* develops a symptom equal to the intensity of the inciting offense.

A rash, though uncomfortable and unsightly, is the most benign symptom that the body can develop. In the hierarchy of organ systems, the skin ranks far below the brain, the heart, and the other internal organs in importance. You can live with an itchy, red rash, but a brain tumor is life threatening. Emily developed a rash in response to a minor grief.

An observant homeopath would recognize what caused Emily's Spiritual Vital Force to be affected, and, instead of giving a cream for the rash, would give a homeopathic remedy designed to restore the Vital Force to its optimal state based on the proving of the indicated remedy. The Vital Force needs something that gives Emily the strength to adapt to her new position in the family. Simply stated, Emily needed a grief remedy.

This brings us to a discussion of something called the *simillimum*. This is the remedy that most closely corresponds to the *totality of symptoms* of a particular case. The goal of the homeopath is to choose the *one* remedy that most closely matches all the symptoms, which is the simillimum. This is akin to having every instrument in the orchestra perfectly in tune and playing at perfect pitch and rhythm.

Oftentimes, a remedy will be *close* to the simillimum, and it will relieve *some* of the client's symptoms. But it is *only* the simillimum that is capable of the *complete annihilation of disease* that restores a person to health. In Emily's case, annihilation of her disease with the correct homeopathic remedy would mean the complete disappearance of *all* of her symptoms: the grief, the rash, the asthma, the ADHD, and the menstrual disorder.

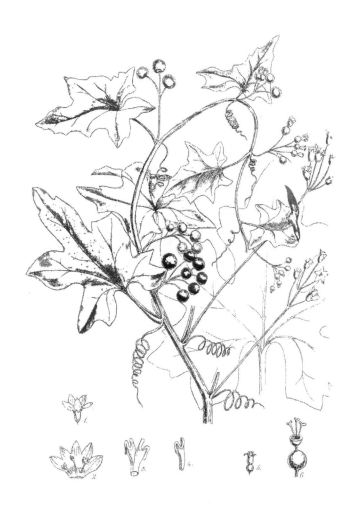

BRYONIA ALBA

CASE STORIES:
Real People, Real Problems

TONI (Depression)

In my own clinic, I have had hundreds of cases with "miraculous" results. One of my most memorable is that of a woman I'll call Toni. When Toni first came to see me, she was suffering from severe suicidal depression after her husband left her for another woman.

Despite being on five psychiatric medications, she still had daily thoughts of suicide. She would fantasize about driving her car off the highest ramp on the freeway or driving it over a cliff. The only reason she hadn't done so was her four-year-old son Sammy, who means everything to her. She felt so guilty that the only thing that was holding her in this world was a small child.

When I took Toni's case, she told me that she had been suicidal since the age of seven. During her entire life, she felt that she had a dark cloud over her head, and she couldn't remember any time when she felt truly happy. Even when Sammy was born, a moment that normally would bring feelings of pure joy, Toni felt numb. She had a very severe form of postpartum depression, and the only thing her psychiatrist could offer was more doses of stronger drugs.

Toni has really high standards for herself and expects everything she does to be perfect. No matter how much her boss praises her for a job well done, she always feels that she could have done better.

This constant self-reproach is a hallmark of a remedy made from gold, called AURUM. In the proving of AURUM, subjects reported feeling severely depressed to the point of suicide. Like Toni, they wanted to jump from a high place like a tall building or throw themselves through windows. This was one of the most striking features of Toni's case. Most women who are suicidal choose a drug overdose. This was such a strong feature in Toni's case that it immediately made me think of AURUM. Her desire for alcohol and general loss of appetite were also characteristic of AURUM.

Toni started with a low potency (6C) of AURUM, nightly. I did not take her off her anti-depressant medications, and this is *critical.* When clients come to me and have been taking prescription medications for any length of time, I have them continue their medications for a while. Medications are like bandages and it is both cruel and inadvisable to remove the protective dressing until the wound has started to heal.

However, Toni felt so horrible on her medications that she stopped three of them within the first month without my knowledge. Fortunately, she felt so much better on the remedy that she had no adverse affects from discontinuing these first three drugs, prematurely in my opinion. Over the next six months, we slowly weaned her off the other two drugs with input from her psychiatrist.

It has been almost six years since Toni started on AURUM. We have gradually increased the potency of the remedy, and she is currently taking AURUM LM60 (a very high potency) daily. She has been on this potency for the past nine months. She is very happy, with a new job and a new boyfriend. She rarely has suicidal thoughts, but when she does, it's a sign that her potency needs changing. Once we increase the potency, her symptoms go away. I anticipate that Toni will need the remedy for another year or so. How will we know when she's finished?

When the remedy has completely annihilated her disease, she will then be healthy, and if she continues to take the remedy, her symptoms will return, and they won't go away with an increase in potency. Continuing to take the remedy would bring on symptoms, as if she were a healthy volunteer in a proving.

Once she stops the remedy, all of her symptoms will go away, and she will be restored to vibrant health, no longer needing medications or even the homeopathic remedy. At some time in the future, if Toni developed a new set of symptoms, she would be re-evaluated, and a new remedy would be chosen.

EMILY, REVISITED

Going back to little Emily, there is a homeopathic remedy

made from a substance in nature that when given to a healthy prover in its crude form produces her symptoms of grief and a red, itchy rash. Instead of giving a drug designed to suppress these symptoms, a homeopath gives her a remedy that matches her set of symptoms. The remedy interacts with the Vital Force. The Vital Force knows exactly how to heal the rash and remove the grief; it just needs a little boost provided by the remedy. As the Vital Force gets stronger, the symptoms gradually disappear without the use of ongoing medications.

In Emily's case, if she had been given the proper homeopathic remedy initially, she would most likely not have developed asthma. The asthma symptoms developed due to a further depletion of the Vital Force. By suppressing the rash with medication, the inciting force (grief) was driven deeper into her being—in this case, into the lungs.

Further suppression with steroids and asthma medication drove the disease even deeper into her nervous system, where she developed symptoms of what conventional medicine calls ADHD. The ADHD drugs caused further suppression of the disease even deeper into her being and this caused the hormonal imbalance. Hence, we see that a lifetime of allopathic suppression not only doesn't heal the original problem but also makes the person sicker and sicker.

What happens if Emily finally gets homeopathic treatment at age fourteen? An observant homeopath assesses what needs to be cured by having a lengthy conversation with Emily and her mother.

During this session, the homeopath's job is to determine the spiritual pattern that has caused her physical symptoms. It is the spiritual Vital Force that "rules the body with unbounded sway," to quote Samuel Hahnemann. Because the Vital Force controls the mind, the body, and the emotions, the task of the homeopath is to understand and identify what Hahnemann called "the morbific influence inimical to life" that caused the symptoms in the first place.

Once this pattern has been identified, a remedy is chosen from the *Materia Medica* and given to the client in a prescribed fashion. As discussed earlier, a remedy can be thought of as analogous to a conductor tuning up an orchestra by directing the musicians to make adjustments in their playing. In a client taking a homeopathic remedy, we begin to see signs of a state of harmony returning.

So, in Emily's case, a remedy is needed that covers all of the symptoms of her disease: grief, asthmatic breathing, attention disorders, and painful menses. As she begins to take the remedy, the most recent symptoms begin to resolve first. In her case, her menstrual pain lessens, her cycles become less heavy, and eventually she is able to stop the birth control pills.

As she continues to heal, her attention span and ability to concentrate improve, and she eventually is weaned off the ADHD medications as well. The grief that she has been harboring since age two begins to abate and finally resolves completely. The rash gets less and less prominent, and, along with the grief, it is the last symptom to completely disappear. In this way, Emily is restored to a state of health, symptom-free and *on no* medications. Eventually the Vital Force is completely healthy, and the remedy is discontinued.

Allopathic medicine is like rearranging the deck chairs on the Titanic. Homeopathy plugs the hole in the boat!

MONA (Allergies, Rash, Fatigue)

When Mona came to see me in December 2010 her skin was a mess. She had moved into a new office the previous year and ever since the move she had a blistery rash over her arms and elbows that "itched like hell and burned like fire". She had seen several skin doctors and had tried a wide variety of creams without any relief.

Besides the rash, she complained of a severe case of fatigue. Despite sleeping ten hours nightly on a CPAP machine for sleep apnea, she would awaken every morning feeling "like I'd been run over by a big truck." During the workday, she would sneak off to her car on her lunch break to take a nap just to be able to finish the afternoon. She bought energy drinks by the case and drank at least two every day.

After hearing her story in detail, I recommended a remedy made from Phosphorous. (Interestingly, her father had built a phosphorous plant in Florida when she was growing up.) She started on the remedy and the results were dramatic. She slept deeply and awakened each morning feeling great. In the first week of taking the remedy, her skin rash got a little worse but by the second week, the itching was dramatically less and she was able to stop using cortisone cream.

Mona is very happy with her progress except for one thing and that's her allergies. In the spring when the Palo Verde trees blossom, her eyes tear up and burn so badly she wants "to take them out of my head and soak them in cold water." Increasing the potency of the Phosphorous didn't help so we added a remedy called Euphrasia, also known as eyebright. She took a dose of 30C and had immediate relief. She continues to take Phosphorous regularly and adds the Euphrasia just when the trees bloom and her eyes react.

Seasonal allergies are a common problem for people all over the country. In the Southwest, people relocate from all over the country and often react to the pollen of unfamiliar desert plants. Many move here from the Midwest and bring a few of their favorite shrubs with them, which cause allergies in Arizona natives who are newly exposed to foreign pollen. The result is lots of itchy eyes, running noses and scratchy throats. There are several remedies for these complaints and we will discuss more of them in the later section on acute remedies.

PEGGY (Food Allergies)

In addition to seasonal allergies, more and more people suffer from food allergies. That turned out to be the culprit in Peggy's case.

Peggy is a bubbly, athletic woman in her late forties who loves to play tennis, run marathons and ride mountain bikes. She's very health conscious and is very careful about her diet. But every morning at 10:00 A.M., almost like clockwork, she has an attack of severe abdominal bloating with gas and diarrhea. Her symptoms are so severe that she has to postpone her morning run until after the attack passes. She takes no medications and has no other symptoms of any kind except for these singular "bowel rebellions".

We drew blood for IgG and IgE antibodies to 150 foods. The only thing she was severely allergic to was egg whites. When I called to give her the results, she practically howled with laughter when I told her. What was the one thing she put in her smoothie every morning for breakfast? You guessed it: two egg whites.

Once she stopped the egg white smoothies, the attacks stopped immediately and she has not had one since. Giving her a remedy would not have helped because the inciting cause was something external, not just a derangement in her Vital Force.

Many, if not most, of the clients I see with diarrhea, constipation, gas or bloating have been give a diagnosis of Irritable Bowel Syndrome and prescribed medications for the symptoms. The first thing I do in these cases is to check them for food allergies. Some will require additional testing for pesticides or preservatives. Once the aggravating factor has been identified, an elimination diet brings relief and the drugs can be stopped.

BECKY and STEFANO (Symptoms: Post-partum fatigue/ Delayed speech development)

Becky is a young mother who recently came to see me for help with a host of symptoms that started two years ago after the birth of her son, Stefano. She had a difficult pregnancy with heart palpitations severe enough that she required medication. Since the delivery, she complains of severe fatigue, exacerbated by the fact that Stefano didn't sleep through the night for the first year. She has noted hair loss by the handfuls as well as an itchy rash on her scalp called seborrheic dermatitis for which she was given a steroid crème and shampoo to use.

Her fatigue has seriously impacted her job by interfering with her ability to concentrate. She would like to go back to school to get her masters in computer science but she's just too tired. After taking her case, we started Becky on a daily dose of SEPIA 6C.

When I saw her for her first follow up after taking the remedy for six weeks, I was actually shocked. She looked like a

36

completely different person and she told me that she hadn't felt this good since high school. She was sleeping better and her hair loss was not as severe. We adjusted her potency and made an appointment to follow up again in six weeks.

She had brought her two-year-old son, Stefano, with her who sat playing a video game on Becky's tablet computer as we spoke. He was healthy looking and obviously very bright but when I spoke to him, he didn't speak back. Becky told me that he had started to say a few words when he was about eleven months old but his speech development stopped completely after he received all his vaccinations at twelve months of age. He would babble and make noise, but he had stopped making words. I gave him one dose of THUJA 30C which is one of the remedies we commonly use for "Ailments after vaccination." (This is such a common problem that there are over 80 remedies used in this condition.)

After a week, Becky called to tell me that on the third day after he received the single dose of the remedy, Stefano began to speak in complete sentences using words they had never heard him speak before.

About two weeks later, Becky called back reporting that Stefano had a fever, excessive drooling and was refusing to eat because his mouth hurt. He was teething as his molars came in. I had Becky give him CHAMOMILLA 30C and the fever, drooling and mouth pain subsided over the next few days. However, the speech problem returned so we repeated the THUJA and he resumed talking. He takes the THUJA about once every few weeks when his speech begins to lag. Eventually his speech should improve permanently and he will no longer need THUJA.

MANDY (Infertility)

Mandy was twenty-six and single when she came to see me in 2003. She had been referred to me by her family physician with the diagnosis of *Premature Ovarian Failure.* She had not had a menses for six months and complained of hot flashes and night sweats that would keep her from getting a good night's sleep. She had seen another gynecologist and hormonal tests revealed her Follicle Stimulating Hormone (FSH) level to be 78; any level greater than 20 is considered menopausal. She was placed on birth control pills, but she began to have nightmares and suicidal thoughts

The birth control pills were discontinued, and she was given Effexor, an anti-depressant medication. When she came to see me, she complained of feeling "emotionally numb."

I spoke with Mandy about using homeopathic treatment to restore her to health by correcting the underlying spiritual cause that was making her sick. I needed her to tell me everything about herself from the time she was a little girl.

She reported to me that she had been sexually abused by her grandfather when she was between seven and fourteen. She told me that she constantly felt torn between two different ways of looking at the world. "One day I'm full of love for the world and for my family, and the next day I could kill the guy who cuts me off in traffic." And just how would she kill him? With a big knife! She said she often felt that she had both "an angel and a devil" inside her.

She told me that when she'd had menses in the past "I think I had the worst case of PMS of anyone in the world. My boyfriend says "PMS" stands for 'Pack My Suitcase,' because I would get so angry he wanted to run away!"

In evaluating Mandy's case, I looked at three rubrics, or symptoms, listed in the *Materia Medica*: Ailments from Abuse, Desire to Kill, and Contradiction of Will.

Searching for all the remedies that have these three traits in common, only two appear, ANACARDIUM ORIENTALE and LYSSINUM. ANACARDIUM is made from a plant and has the very prominent symptom that Mandy expressed: "Delusion that a demon and an angel sit on his shoulders telling him offensive or good things."

ANACARDIUM is also indicated in cases of manic depression.

LYSSINUM, which is made from rabies, is associated with a profound fear of water, which she did not have. ANACARDIUM best covered the entire case.

I started Mandy on ANACARDIUM 6C daily. At her first follow-up visit six weeks later, she reported that she was much less irritable and depressed. We adjusted the potency and agreed to meet again in 6 weeks.

Twelve weeks after starting the remedy, she reported that she had a menstrual period but reported no symptoms of PMS. Over the course of a year, we gradually increased the potency of the remedy as we slowly lowered the dose of the Effexor. She became engaged to be married and reported that she was "very happy."

Three years after starting Homeopathy, Mandy gave birth to a healthy baby girl. For someone who had been told that she had premature menopause and would never have a child, Homeopathy was truly a blessing. This is just one of the "miracles" that we see everyday with Homeopathy.

CRYSTAL (Chronic Headaches)

Crystal was twenty-four when she came to see me in the spring of 2008 complaining that she wasn't having menstrual cycles. She had a complicated history for someone so young. As a child, she had recurrent ear infections and sinus infections from the age of six for which she was given multiple courses of antibiotics. In addition, she had a mild scoliosis and had her spine X rayed every four months until she was sixteen.

At the age of nine she developed severe depression and she was placed on anti-depressant therapy. She would frequently have severe bouts of flu where she would become dehydrated from vomiting.

When Crystal reached the usual age of puberty, she didn't start her menses as expected and started having headaches that were so painful, she would miss school. A thorough evaluation by her pediatrician showed abnormal hair growth on her abdomen, high levels of testosterone in her blood and multiple cysts on her ovaries. She was given the diagnosis of *Polycystic Ovarian Syndrome* and started on birth control pills. This made her headaches much worse and when she stopped the pills, the menses she had while taking them stopped.

In addition, she had severe fatigue and was placed on thyroid medication.

Homeopathic consultation and evaluation of her entire case including her dreams and food preferences indicated a remedy called CALCAREA PHOSPHORICA. She started the remedy in April and within 4 months she had her first menses. Over the past 4 years with ongoing adjustments in her remedy potencies, she now has regular monthly menses and the only time she has headaches is when her remedy needs adjusting.

Homeopathy can be used not only for chronic conditions but it is a very powerful, often life-saving tool in the case of serious illnesses and emergencies.

BETH (Acute Appendicitis)

Several years ago, I received a phone call one morning from the emergency department of my local hospital. The physician on duty told me that one of my clients had been in his department since 3:00 A.M. with acute abdominal pain. She had a high fever, an elevated white blood cell count, and the abdominal CT scan showed acute appendicitis. The surgeon on call had been in to see her and recommended immediate surgery. However, she had no health insurance and didn't like the surgeon, who had scolded her for getting him up in the middle of the night.

She was threatening to leave against medical advice, and the physician on duty asked if I would see her. I agreed, and her husband drove her to my office. As she walked in, I could see that she was in severe pain. She told me that the pain was especially severe when she moved.

The slightest touch to her abdomen brought on excruciating pain. She had rebound tenderness on palpation, a hallmark of acute appendicitis. I discussed homeopathic treatment with her and her husband, with the understanding that if she did not show improvement within thirty minutes, I would admit her to the hospital and perform an appendectomy.

With their permission, I gave her one dose of BRYONIA 200C while she was lying on the examination table with a thermometer in her mouth. She immediately fell asleep, and her temperature began to drop—from 102.3°F to 100.0°F within a half hour.

As she slept, I was able to gently palpate her abdomen without awakening her. After sleeping for about three hours, she awakened with a normal temperature and said that her pain was only half as intense as it had been before taking the remedy. We repeated the dose, and she went back to sleep. At 6:00 P.M., after receiving a total of four doses of BRYONIA 200C, she woke up pain-free and hungry. I sent her home with more of the remedy and my home phone number.

I had her husband call me when she woke up during the night (twice), and the remedy was given again each time. When she called me the next morning, she said that she was completely pain-free and had just taken her dogs for a walk. Such an outcome is not uncommon if the correct homeopathic remedy is chosen and given frequently enough and in the correct potency.

In Beth's case, BRYONIA saved the woman from having to undergo an operation. As far as I know, she still has her appendix. A word of caution here: BRYONIA is NOT the only remedy used to treat acute appendicitis. Each case is unique and may require a different remedy. There are other remedies for acute appendicitis when the patient is restless and thrashing around with pain.

In Beth's case the hallmark symptom that indicated BRYONIA was the necessary remedy was her aversion to movement. Everything was worse when she moved and this is the *sine qua non* of BRYONIA. BRYONIA is also indicated when the patient holds his or her belly tightly to obtain some relief by applying deep pressure.

Obviously another person with acute appendicitis, who is writhing on the bed in pain, needs a different remedy where RESTLESSNESS WITH PAIN is the key symptom. Giving this person BRYONIA would have no effect.

EMERGENCY SITUATIONS (CHELSEA)

Life often deals us the unexpected, and in the course of homeopathic treatment clients sometimes experience acute symptoms. These may arise from outside influences such as accidents. But often, acute situations are actually the returning of old symptoms that were suppressed for years.

Chelsea is an example of the latter situation. She is a beautiful, hardworking physical therapist who first came to me about three years ago for help with a severe rash that plagued her off and on for years. She had a history of recurrent ear infections as a child, for which she was given very frequent courses of antibiotics. She also had asthma as a child; it was so severe, she required steroid treatment, which caused a lot of weight gain that became a focus of concern in the family. She was often deprived of things she wanted unless she lost weight.

In her twenties, Chelsea often participated in pharmaceutical drug trials to help support herself while in college. During a study of an immunosuppressive drug, she had a severe reaction that caused a massive case of hives. To this day, she gets hives if she takes certain commonly used drugs, such as Tylenol.

When I took Chelsea's case, she reported to me that she frequently had dreams of flying since childhood, and that she was currently estranged from her mother and brother due to conflict over her grandmother's will. The resulting litigation was very distressing to Chelsea. Also, she reported that she loved to dance and did it a lot. The remedy I chose for Chelsea was POSITRONIUM, which is prepared from the radiation arising from the annihilation of POSITRONIUM atoms. A remedy can be made from anything God created which includes everything in the Universe. I learned about this remedy from Vega Rozenberg at an ESSH seminar in 2008.

We started with a 6C every other day because of Chelsea's skin condition. Often times, the skin will aggravate when beginning a remedy and the rash can become quite severe, so we started slowly. Over the past three years, Chelsea has improved dramatically.

Last fall, Chelsea called with complaints of a sore throat, fever, and aching all over. Her fever would spike as high as 104°F, and then she'd have shaking chills. She complained of severe neck pain. When I examined her she didn't have the rigidity in the neck that is the hallmark of meningitis.

The homeopath in me knew that this was the effect of three years of a good remedy pushing out all of the disease that had been suppressed ever since childhood, as well as the effects of her participation in the pharmaceutical trials.

Over the course of ten days, Chelsea required multiple remedies repeated frequently. After four remedies repeated hourly for 36 hours, her fever broke, the muscle aches resolved, and the severe fatigue began to lift.

The allopath in me knew that if she had gone to the Emergency Room, they would have done a spinal tap, and she would have been given the diagnosis of aseptic spinal meningitis.

At her last follow-up, Chelsea reported that she has never felt better in her entire life. When the Vital Force goes through such a healing crisis, it invariably comes out stronger on the other side. Chelsea had the stamina and fortitude to stick with the remedies, even though there were many times when she was tempted to take allopathic drugs. If the symptoms were suppressed again, her overall health would deteriorate and put her at risk for some more deadly disease in the future.

Time will tell how much longer she is going to need the POSITRONIUM, but for now she looks and feels great. The rash is completely gone and rarely comes back. The litigation with her family has been resolved, and she is at peace.

Sometimes, when a person develops new symptoms, just increasing the frequency or the potency of his or her "constitutional" remedy will be enough. This is the first thing to try, and it is what I did with Chelsea. However, if the client doesn't respond significantly after a few doses, then the Vital Force needs something else added. Usually a single remedy is enough. But when clients with a longstanding illness become acutely sick, several remedies might need to be repeated frequently over several days, always using their symptoms as a guide to the proper choice of remedy.

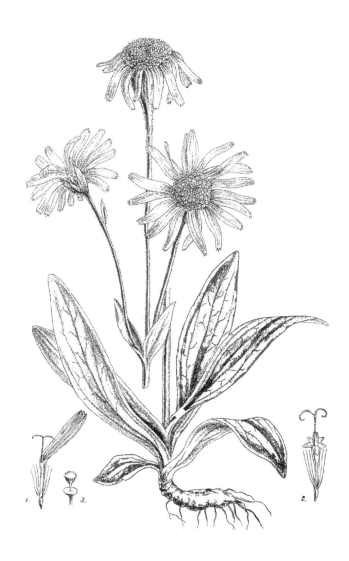

ARNICA MONTANA

FREQUENTLY ASKED QUESTIONS

WHY ISN'T HOMEOPATHY "MAINSTREAM"?

If Homeopathy works so well, why isn't it more widely used today in the U.S.? Up until the early 1900s, about a third of American physicians were homeopaths, and about a third of American hospitals were homeopathic. The physicians who founded the American Medical Association (AMA) were aligned with the patent medicine companies, the forerunners of the modern pharmaceutical companies.

There was intense competition for patients between physicians who prescribed patent drugs and homeopaths who used remedies. Members of the AMA were not allowed to collaborate or socialize with homeopaths. Physicians who were not AMA members were not allowed to admit patients to hospitals.

The result: Homeopathy was rendered virtually extinct in America by interfering with the ability of homeopaths to make a living. The best source of information about this sad phenomenon is Harris Coulter's book, *Divided Legacy*. [See REFRENCES.]

Despite being blackballed by the medical establishment, Homeopathy in America has persisted. In other parts of the world, it has continued to grow and thrive since Hahnemann's day. Personally, I think Homeopathy manages to survive here because it is the truest form of healing, and the truth can't be completely suppressed.

We are currently seeing a resurgence of interest in Homeopathy because of the failings of conventional, allopathic medicine, which does *not* restore people to a place of health but merely "shoots the messenger" by falsely equating symptoms with disease. The *truth* is that disease is a disordered state of the Vital Force, and symptoms are merely warning signs.

One of the most serious failings of conventional, allopathic medicine is the development of various forms of bacteria such as MRSA (Methicillin Resistant *Staphylococcus aureus*) and antibiotic resistant strains of Tuberculosis and Gonorrhea. Homeopathy can be a lifesaver in treating these conditions where conventional therapies have ceased to work. Addressing the disruption of the client's Vital Force and choosing the appropriate remedy based on the totality of symptoms can restore them to health, even in life threatening circumstances.

HOW DOES HOMEOPATHY DIFFER FROM NATUROPATHY AND HERBAL MEDICINE?

Homeopathy is a specific form of healing that works on the Spiritual Vital Force. Naturopathic medicine uses nutrition, herbs and, in some states, pharmaceutical drugs to treat the physical body. Although there is some education about Homeopathy in Naturopathic schools, in my experience most Naturopaths who become Homeopaths do so only after further education, because the number of hours of Homeopathic training in Naturopathic schools is limited.

IS HOMEOPATHY JUST THE PLACEBO EFFECT?

The placebo effect occurs when people believe they are better after taking a substance that they think has medicinal properties but is actually non-medicinal, such as a pill containing only sugar. We know that Homeopathy is not a placebo because it works for infants, animals, and even in the comatose or unconscious. A placebo will not stop bleeding or eliminate a high fever, but a properly chosen Homeopathic remedy will.

HOW DO I FIND A QUALIFIED HOMEOPATH

How does one go about finding a homeopath who consistently gets good results? Unfortunately, this is a problem, especially in the U.S., where there are all kinds of perversions of principles done in the name of Homeopathy.

The first question to have answered is whether your prospective homeopath does Homeopathy in the same way that Hahnemann taught it. This means having a clear understanding of the *spiritual nature* of Homeopathy as Hahnemann first described it in the *Organon of Medicine* and as one of my teachers, Vega Rozenberg has strongly emphasized in his teachings today.

The most effective homeopaths evaluate the *totality of symptoms* and have a good understanding of what has disrupted the spiritual vital force. Giving one remedy for a sore throat, another for the cough and yet another for fever is allopathic, not homeopathic. Understanding the spiritual pattern present that indicates *the one* remedy that adjusts the Vital Force avoids much mischief and will successfully achieve the goal of ANNIHILATING the disease rather than just suppressing symptoms.

In rare (generally acute) cases, more than one remedy is required, but the basic principle of understanding the spiritual pattern underlying the disease still holds true. Recalling the orchestra analogy, it is impossible to play a beautiful symphony on the stage of Carnegie Hall if there's a brass band playing in the lobby and a rock band blaring from the balcony.

Another sign that your practitioner is not following closely in the path of Hahnemann is if he or she uses a machine applied to the skin to tell which remedies are needed. This usually results in the prescription of several remedies all at once. Oftentimes this deranges the vital force so much that the client actually becomes sicker.

Unfortunately, I have seen many cases of people developing serious, life-threatening illnesses when treated in this way.

Find out where your prospective practitioner trained and how many years of training they have had. A medical doctor with only ninety hours of training in Homeopathy is very unlikely to know how to use the more than 5,000 remedies we currently have in our Materia Medica.

If possible, talk to other clients of the prospective practitioner and determine whether or not they have had curative results. A successful homeopath treats clients so effectively that they don't need to come back after a course of treatment unless something else deranges the state of good health to which Homeopathy restores them.

How does the homeopath know which disease is present that needs to be annihilated? By taking a thorough inventory of the life of the client and gathering the *totality* of symptoms. This is called "taking the case."

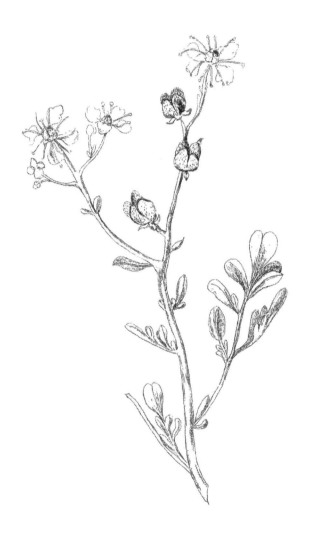

RUTA GRAVEOLENS

THE HOMEOPATHIC PROCESS

CASE TAKING

I think it is helpful for my clients to have some understanding of the kinds of information a good homeopath needs in order to choose the simillimum. Ascertaining the simillimum is not possible without taking a good case. Taking a case is a special skill; it is actually the *foundation* of the Art of Homeopathy.

Without a clear picture of the disease that needs to be removed it is impossible for the homeopath to choose the simillimum correctly.

The first step in taking the case, also known as the homeopathic interview, occurs long before the homeopath and the client actually meet. As Vega Rozenberg has emphasized in his lectures at ESSH on numerous occasions, in order to understand what is abnormal, or disturbed in a person, a homeopath must first understand what is normal. This is why medical students begin their training with anatomy. In order to recognize a pancreas damaged from cancer, for example, one must know what a healthy pancreas looks like. Similarly, a homeopath must have a good understanding of human nature in order to see what circumstances and conditions have caused the client's Vital Force to become unbalanced.

CASE ANALYSIS

Once the homeopath has taken the case and gathered all of the client's symptoms, his/her job is to choose the *one* remedy that, when given correctly and adjusted over time, will successfully annihilate the disease and restore the person to health. This is called *evaluating the case*. This is quite a challenge, since there are more than 5,000 remedies catalogued in the *Materia Medica*. In analyzing a case, the homeopath uses a *Repertory*, which is a catalog of all the symptoms of all of the remedies in the *Materia*

Medica. These symptoms are organized in sections that correspond to the anatomy of the human body.

Prior to the invention of computers, case analysis was done by hand. I remember evaluating my first cases using *Kent's Repertory* and large pieces of graph paper. It was tedious and time consuming. Fortunately, a gifted gentleman named David Warkentin, of blessed memory, devised a computer program called *MacRepertory.* This has changed the lives of most every homeopath working today—now that Mac*Repertory* and the *Materia Medica* known as ReferenceWorks are literally at our fingertips.

I think that if it were not for David and his elegant computer programs, most of us would have given up on Homeopathy out of sheer frustration due to the tedium of case analysis. Though David has since passed on, his legacy remains, and I am just one of a multitude of homeopaths and their clients grateful to him for the benefits we have received from his life's work. Thank you, David, wherever you are.

Let's briefly review how a homeopath uses the *Repertory* and the *Materia Medica* to evaluate a case.

For example, in evaluating an acute case of nausea the homeopath refers to the section of the *Repertory* corresponding to the stomach: *"Stomach, Nausea".* There are **884** remedies listed, which is not very helpful. However, if the client also has nausea with the urge to vomit, the rubric *"Stomach,* Nausea, vomiting, desire to,"* is more helpful and has only thirty-three remedies. In looking closely at this rubric, we see one remedy that is capitalized, in bold type, and underlined.

This remedy is NUX-V (NUX VOMICA). When a remedy is so prominently displayed, it means that the symptom of *nausea with an urge to vomit* is a very characteristic symptom of this remedy that was reported by a large proportion of the volunteers who took NUX VOMICA in the proving.

Other remedies listed include Phos (PHOSPHORUS) and Ars (ARSENICUM). Distinguishing between these three remedies requires a thorough knowledge of each of the remedies.

NUX VOMICA, for example, is a remedy often indicated for

overworked businessmen with hangovers following excessive alcohol intake. So, it's important in this case to ask the client if their symptoms came on after they went on a bender.

If that is not the case, then further investigation is needed. ARSENICUM is the most common remedy for cases of acute food poisoning, often accompanied by diarrhea and severe chills. If the client reports that these concomitant symptoms came on after eating tuna salad at a picnic, then ARSENICUM is the likely *simillimum*.

If the client denies the above but complains of nausea that comes on after drinking warm liquids and they complain of feeling "wiped out", PHOSPHORUS is the more likely choice.

POTENCY

Once the homeopath has determined the correct remedy, how does he or she decide what potency to recommend and how often to give it? As a general rule, in acute cases the 30C potency is the best choice. How often the remedy is repeated depends on the strength of the symptoms.

A few years back, I had a severe case of food poisoning after eating lunch at a popular salad buffet restaurant. Within forty-five minutes, I had a full-blown attack of all the symptoms associated with food poisoning. Without being too graphic, I'll note that the symptoms were so severe that my assistant had to drive me home (where the remedy was) while I was vomiting into a wastebasket.

The chills were so bad that my teeth chattered. The first dose of ARSENICUM 30C increased the retching. I phoned my homeopath and he had me repeat the remedy every fifteen minutes for the first one and a half hours.

Each time I repeated the dose, the retching got worse. This was my body's way of getting rid of the "morbific agent inimical to life" that was served with my salad. After ninety minutes the vomiting stopped, but the nausea persisted. I continued to take the remedy every thirty minutes for the next two hours.

Gradually, as the symptoms subsided, I needed the remedy less often. I took two doses during the night, and when I awoke in the morning, I was perfectly well and able to go to work, where I saw a full day's worth of clients.

I took a dose or two each day for the next three days just to make sure the "morbific agent" that made me sick was completely gone. All of the symptoms I had were consistent with *Salmonella* poisoning.

If I had gone to my hospital Emergency Room, I would have been given intravenous antibiotics and fluids and probably admitted to the hospital for two or three days.

This example demonstrates how important it is to repeat the remedy frequently enough to assist the Vital Force in making a complete and rapid recovery possible. If the proper remedy is not given with adequate potency, frequency, and duration, a chronic condition can ensue. This often happens in cases of food poisoning that are not treated homeopathically.

Fatigue is often one of the symptoms that can persist after a bout with *Salmonella*. Many times it takes people weeks or even months to recover. Some unfortunate people never fully recover, and a case of *Chronic Fatigue Syndrome* ensues. Allopathic medicine fails to see the connection and considers *Chronic Fatigue Syndrome* just another set of symptoms that randomly occur for no reason.

However, in Homeopathy it is understood that the cause of illness is something deeper than a bad tango with a nasty bacterium named *Salmonella*. We understand that there is a *spirit-like morbific influence* that causes physical and sometimes emotional symptoms. (During my bout of food poisoning, I really did have a fear that I would die, which is a hallmark of ARSENICUM and one of the symptoms that led me to choose it over other remedies that work for food poisoning.)

If we fail to completely eradicate the morbific influence inimical to life, then we have not succeeded in annihilating the disease. Consequently, the person will continue to suffer, and the condition will evolve into something like Chronic Fatigue Syndrome.

WHAT TO EXPECT FROM TREATMENT

Once the homeopath has taken the case and determined the proper remedy, how is the remedy given and when are changes made? Entire books and articles have been written on this subject since Hahnemann's day. Some homeopaths prefer to use high potencies infrequently while others use low potencies frequently and repeat them over time. The finer details of this debate are beyond the scope of this book. Your homeopath will instruct you regarding the potency and the frequency of the remedy.

When the remedy has been taken for a period of time, a follow up discussion is scheduled to assess the effect of the remedy. When a person begins taking a remedy, his/her Vital Force starts to become stronger and healthier—the orchestra begins to come back into tune. As the remedy interacts with the Spiritual Vital Force, it's as if each instrument in the orchestra becomes more precise and brilliant in its sound. The entire orchestra is now playing in harmony. Similarly, the symptoms that were an indicator of disharmony or disease in the body begin to abate. This state of harmony may be permanent or it may persist for a period of time and then begin to fade. As the symptoms begin to return, adjustments in potency and frequency need to be made. Each time the symptoms return, it is as if the conductor is asking for a change in pitch, volume or rhythm depending on what's needed to restore harmony. In this way, a homeopath learns to "listen" to the messages sent from the Vital Force and make the appropriate changes.

A word about something called a Homeopathic *aggravation* is appropriate here. As the Vital Force begins to respond to the remedy, sometimes symptoms will worsen. This is usually an indication that the remedy is working. Adjusting the frequency of the potency is usually enough to manage the aggravation and your homeopath can make recommendations to help you through what some people call a "healing crisis." Once the aggravation passes, the frequency of the remedy is usually adjusted to a more regular schedule.

HOW LONG WILL HOMEOPATHIC TREATMENT TAKE?

Clients often ask how long this process takes. The true answer to this question is "Only God knows." Homeopathic healing is a process that takes time and will vary from one person to another.

A general rule of thumb is that the longer one has had an illness, the longer the time of treatment required.

I often remind my clients that they didn't get sick overnight, and the curative process takes time and patience. Of course, in acute or emergency situations, the result is often immediate, and the condition resolves over hours or days instead of months or years. Generally, the longer one has had an illness, the longer the time of treatment required.

DURING HOMEOPATHIC TREATMENT, SHOULD I STOP TAKING MY OTHER MEDICATIONS?

In a word, "No." I advise my clients to continue their medications and to take the remedy at least two hours after their medicines. As I described earlier, medications are like bandages and we don't peel off the dressing until the wound has started to heal. As the Vital Force becomes stronger, the symptoms for which the medications were prescribed will begin to dissipate. Clients are then slowly weaned off their pharmaceutical drugs over time with the assistance of their physicians.

Recently, while I was a guest on a radio show, I took a call from a woman who told me that she had been a Type I insulin dependent diabetic since childhood. She recently consulted a naturopath who told her to stop her insulin! Fortunately, she was educated enough to know that this was deadly advice.

IS THERE ANYTHING THAT WILL INTERFERE WITH THE REMEDY?

Yes. Coffee and strong mint halt the action of homeopathic remedies. This is known as antidoting. Decaf coffee does the same thing. It is not the caffeine in these drinks that disrupts the process. Rather, it is the energetic signatures of coffee and mint that interfere with the healing action of homeopathic remedies

HOW WILL I KNOW WHEN I AM DONE
WITH THE REMEDY?

Remember that the fundamental principle of Homeopathy is that *like heals like*: a substance given to healthy people brings on a set of symptoms in a process known as a proving. When a remedy made from this substance is given to an ill person with the same symptoms, the Spiritual Vital Force is strengthened, restoring the person to health.

Once health is restored, the person no longer needs the remedy. If he/she continues to take the remedy when healthy, the symptoms will come back, because he/she is now "proving" the remedy; after the remedy is stopped, the symptoms will go away. A well-trained Homeopath will recognize when a person is healthy, and the remedy needs to be stopped.

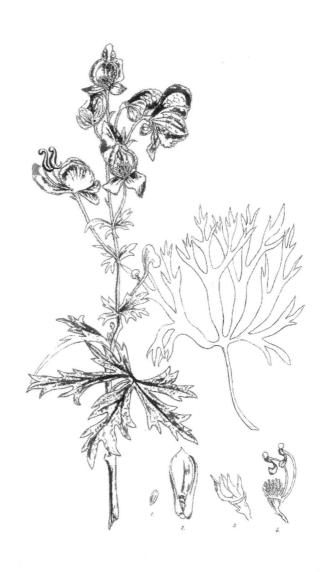

ACONITUM NAPELLUS

DO IT YOURSELF: EMERGENCY AND ACUTE HOMEOPATHIC CARE

Now that you have a basic understanding of how Homeopathy works, how can you go about using it to benefit yourself and others? Just as in cases of chronic illness, traumatic events that we think of as "accidents" have a basis in spirit.

A traumatic event occurs because the spiritual Vital Force has been attacked. When a properly chosen homeopathic remedy is given, the spiritual vital force is stimulated to "fight back" and hence is restored to its state of health. Because the spiritual vital force controls every function of the body, physical, mental and emotional health ensues. It is only by affecting the spiritual Vital Force that the body, mind, and emotions of a person are brought back into harmony.

9/11

I have a close friend who has a corner office in the World Financial Center, the building that sits adjacent to the former site of the World Trade Center, also known as "Ground Zero." On that Tuesday in September 2001, he was an eye-witness to a scene of carnage that is usually only seen in a war zone. At first unable to leave his building, his senses were bombarded as he witnessed the deaths of thousands. Thank God he and his co-workers eventually were allowed to leave the building.

Covered in dust from the falling towers, he walked several miles through the streets of lower Manhattan with thousands of other panicked New Yorkers. Not previously anxious, soon thereafter he began feeling anxiety and had difficulty sleeping. Homeopathic ACONITE 30C nightly for about a week was enough to relieve his symptoms.

Soldiers returning from war who suffer from *Post-Traumatic Stress Disorder* are often in a chronic ACONITE state, characterized by anxiety, insomnia, nightmares, and difficulty concentrating. Homeopathic treatment with ACONITE would work wonders for these brave men and women who serve so stoically, yet suffer so much.

DOING IT YOURSELF

One of the best ways to acquaint yourself with the power of Homeopathy is to get an Emergency Kit and try it on yourself and your family members for cases of acute illness. The following is a general guide to the most common emergencies or acute conditions encountered, especially if you have children.

This is not meant to be a substitute for homeopathic *consultation.* It is a basic introduction that will help to guide you when you are standing in front of a display of homeopathic remedies at a health food store, wondering what to buy when you have a cold or the beginnings of the flu.

For more serious or chronic illnesses, consult a homeopathic professional, as discussed above.

The second thing you will need is a Home Remedy Kit. I recommend that my clients purchase theirs from Hahnemann Homeopathic Pharmacy because I am familiar with their Kits [See RESOURCES].

The HHP Home Remedy Kit contains 50 remedies and costs around $135.00. This kit will last a long time as long as it is properly stored and does not come into contact with Xrays or microwaves.

Additional homeopathic pharmacies are listed in the RESOURCES SECTION.

HOMEOPATHIC TREATMENT FOR COMMON AILMENTS

I have chosen the following remedies as they are the ones most commonly available to the general public in health food stores.

These remedies can be used for a wide variety of conditions and form the basis of a Home Remedy Kit.

As a general rule, when using homeopathic remedies in acute illnesses, start with the 30C potency and repeat it as needed depending on the response. In situations of severe symptoms, the remedy can be repeated every fifteen minutes until the symptoms begin to abate. Then gradually decrease how often the remedy is given as things return to normalcy. For a detailed description of such a case, see the discussion on Food Poisoning in the previous section.

ALLERGIES AND HAY FEVER

These symptoms are so common that I would say up to 40% of the clients I see are on some kind of nasal spray or decongestant, depending on the seasons. Clients with longstanding allergies that have been suppressed for years by allergy injections or chronic medications will usually require *constitutional* treatment in order to restore their Vital Force to a state of health.

For people with *acute hay fever* who have not had years of conventional, suppressive medications, a few remedies can bring immediate relief of annoying symptoms without the side effects common with pharmaceutical drugs.

For clients who are already on a constitutional remedy and develop allergies, the first thing to do is to try increasing the frequency or the potency of their remedy. If this does not bring relief, then they need a course of an acute remedy consistent with their symptoms.

ALLIUM CEPA, made from red onion, is the remedy of choice for *hay fever* or *colds* with the primary symptom of *extreme tearing*. If you have ever chopped a raw onion and had tears running down your face, you'll know the symptoms that indicate you need ALLIUM CEPA.

When *itching of the eyes* is the primary symptom, EUPHRASIA is indicated. The *sensation of sand in the eyes* is a hallmark of EUPHRASIA.

HEPAR SULPHURIS CALCAREUM (HEPAR) is indicated in cases of *severe sore throat* with *chills*. It's also very helpful for *seasonal allergies* where the main symptom is a very sore throat.

ARSENICUM ALBUM is the remedy to use when there is marked sneezing, itching of the soft palate, and asthma.

CARBO VEGETABILIS is often indicated in cases of *asthma* with sore throat and sneezing. The hallmarks of CARBO VEGETABILIS are *air hunger and a desire to be fanned.*

DULCAMARA is the remedy to consider when *hay fever* strikes and the client is *better from warm applications* to the nose and worse from being in cold air.

COLDS AND FLU

Nothing makes a person more convinced of the power of Homeopathy then to recover successfully and quickly from an acute illness that would normally drag on for days.

While allopathic medicine focuses on suppressing symptoms, homeopathy is designed to restore the weakened Vital Force to a state of health. There are several remedies indicated for colds and flu and, as is true for any condition, the choice of remedy is dictated by the constellation of symptoms.

The first remedy to think of at the onset of any inflammatory or febrile condition is FERRUM PHOSPHORICUM. This remedy doesn't have the sudden onset of such remedies as ACONITE or BELLADONNA, but it acts faster than GELSEMIUM. The typical case that warrants FERRUM PHOSPHORICUM is that of a person who catches colds easily. The first symptoms are usually a sore throat, a pale yet easily flushed face, and a marked feeling of weakness—the person just doesn't feel like getting out of bed.

Taking FERRUM PHOSPHORICUM at the first sign of a cold will often stop or shorten the usual progression of a cold.

ACONITE is the remedy to give when the cold symptoms

come on suddenly after exposure to cold weather and especially dry, cold wind or air conditioning. There is usually a feeling of marked anxiety, and the chills can feel as if they penetrate right to the bone. People needing ACONITE tend to be very restless and alternate between bed and sofa when they are ill.

GELSEMIUM is the remedy to think of when people complain of severe weakness and drowsiness with the onset of a cold or flu. They tend to ache all over, and their muscles feel so weak they are sore. They appear apathetic and dull, and their mental functions are sluggish. In chronic cases, people will report that they have "never been well since the flu." A good course of GELSEMIUM has been known to cure long-standing cases of Chronic Fatigue Syndrome that started after a bout of the flu.

DROSERA ROTUNDIFOLIA is the remedy of choice for someone with a deep, whooping cough. The cough is spasmodic and often has a barking quality to it. Victims try their best to bring up a bit of phlegm, but this usually leads to vomiting.

The cough tends to worsen at night and often leads to hoarseness. Sometimes the coughing and vomiting are so severe that there is bleeding from the nose or coughing up of blood. Persons needing DROSERA tend to be moody, irritable, and stubborn. They are also very restless and can't seem to focus their attention on one thing.

BAPTISIA TINCTORIA, made from wild indigo, is an important remedy in cases of epidemic influenza when almost everyone is sick. Clients needing this remedy often have sleepy expressions on their faces and complain of feeling "sick all over."

Symptoms typically include a high fever, a headache in the forehead and the root of the nose and a sinking sensation in the stomach. Sufferers tend to be restless and move around in bed.

Sleeplessness is a common complaint of those who need BAPTISIA. It's the first remedy to think of in cases of the *mumps*. BAPTISIA is also a remedy that is helpful for problems that arise *after vaccination.*

THUJA is the other remedy to consider when there has been a reaction to vaccination.

SPONGIA TOSTA is the classic remedy to consider for the annoying, dry cough that starts with a "tickle" in the throat. The hallmark of this remedy is the feeling of being "dry as a bone" with dry mucus membranes. Like ACONITE, this remedy is needed for coughing that comes on after exposure to a dry, cold wind, and it is the remedy to consider when ACONITE doesn't completely relieve such symptoms. Gland swelling and thyroid disorders also respond well to SPONGIA.

Colds or flu with severe bone pain call for EUPATORIUM PERFOLATIUM. The pain in the bones can be so severe it feels as if the bones were broken. This remedy is very helpful in cases of *Dengue Fever* where deep bone pain is common.

A *wet, "rattling" cough* in cases of bronchitis or pneumonia calls for ANTIMONIUM TARTARICUM. When this remedy is needed, large amounts of mucus accumulate but very little is expectorated. ANTIMONIUM TARTARICUM helps to expel the mucus that accumulates in the bronchial tubes or deeper in the lung. This remedy should not be confused with its cousin ANTIMONIUM CRUDUM that is more commonly used for disorders of the gastrointestinal tract.

CARBO VEGETABILIS is commonly used for colds, bronchitis or asthma where there is significant *air hunger*, where the person feels they can't catch their breath.

ACUTE INFECTIONS and ABSCESSES

In cases of acute infections, it's important to treat the underlying cause as well as the effects of infection. In allopathic medicine, the emphasis is on determining which bacteria is causing the infection and then prescribing an antibiotic to kill the offending organism.

In Homeopathy, the approach is different. We understand

that the Vital Force is under attack and that the immune system has been overwhelmed. The Vital Force lacks the ability to fight off the infection alone and needs help. By paying close attention to the symptoms, the proper remedy can be chosen which strengthens the Vital Force and allows it to properly guide the immune system to restore the person to a state of health.

For example, if someone develops an abscess after an insect bite, and if the wound is red, hot and inflamed, give APIS. For the secondary infection, adding PYROGENIUM will help the Vital Force remove the infection.

I find PYROGENIUM to be more effective than antibiotics in that it works more quickly and often avoids a long course of pharmaceutical drug treatment.

PYROGENIUM is especially helpful for abscessed teeth or post-operative infections. Any time there is pus present, PYROGENIUM is usually the remedy of choice. If it's early in the process, start with the 30C potency. If the abscess is well developed and the person has had it for several days, start with 200C.

The remedy usually needs to be repeated frequently at the onset, then less frequently as the infection subsides. PYROGENIUM will often facilitate the draining of pus in an abscess and avoid the need for surgical drainage.

SINUS INFECTIONS

These are common infections that often plague people whose Vital Force has become weakened from allergies or exposure to toxic chemicals.

KALI BICHROMICUM is the first remedy to consider when there is *thick, stringy, green discharge*. Oftentimes, this sticky mucus fills the sinus cavities and instead of draining causes a build up of pressure over the cheekbones that can be very painful. Taking KALI BICHROMICUM allows the sinuses to drain and the pressure to be relieved. Clients will frequently call me after they have started this remedy alarmed about the amount of mucus discharge coming from the nose and down the back of the throat. I reassure them that this is a sign of healing.

In fact, if the sinuses DON'T DRAIN after taking KALI BICHROMICUM then another remedy is indicated. A close cousin to this remedy is KALI CARBONICUM. Clients needing this remedy will often have a *sinus infection progressing to bronchitis.* They also tend to have *sweating and cold intolerance.*

KALI SULPHURATUM is a closely related remedy where there is a large amount of deep yellow discharge that may be thin or sticky. Typically, the person needing this remedy feels *hot and irritable.*

URINARY TRACT INFECTIONS

In the healthy state, the urine in the bladder is sterile, meaning that it is free of bacteria. When the immune system fails to function properly, bacteria travel into the bladder and cause an inflammatory response. Typical symptoms of a bladder infection include the urge to urinate frequently, often with very little urine released.

There is usually pain with urination and sometimes blood is seen in the urine. The choice of the proper remedy is dependent on the symptoms and the circumstances under which they arose.

CANTHARIS, made from Spanish Fly, is the remedy of choice when these symptoms come on after a romantic weekend where there is a lot of intercourse. Typically clients will complain that the pain comes at the *end of urination.*

STAPHYSAGRIA is another very common remedy indicated in cases of *frequently recurring bladder infections,* especially *after catheterization.*

BERBERIS VULGARIS is called for if there is *flank pain over the kidneys.* It is the first remedy to think of in case of *kidney stones.* BERBERIS is also helpful for *gallstone colic with jaundice* but serious conditions involving jaundice (yellowing of the skin) indicate liver blockage and require professional care.

MERCURIUS SOLUBULIS HAHNEMANN (MERCURIUS) is very helpful for urinary conditions where there is a strong urge to urinate. There is often *incontinence or involuntary bedwetting.* When a person needs MERCURIUS, there can also be *drooling during sleep* and an acute *sensitivity to temperature.*

FOOD POISONING

The dramatic response to Homeopathic treatment of food poisoning has turned many a skeptic into a believer in the power of Homeopathy.

ARSENICUM ALBUM is the remedy indicated when the symptoms include *nausea, vomiting, chills and desire to drink in small sips.* VERATRUM ALBUM may also be used for these same symptoms but the person needling ARSENICUM will often have anxiety and a fear that they might die.

They also will tend to drink larger quantities at a time instead of sipping. In my experience, the most common mistake people make when using Homeopathy for food poisoning is that they don't take the remedy frequently enough and often stop it prematurely. At the onset of symptoms, the remedy may need to be given every fifteen minutes.

As the symptoms abate, the remedy is given less often. It should be continued for two to three days after all the symptoms are gone in order to prevent the Vital Force from weakening again and the symptoms returning. [See pp. 53-54]

CHINA OFFICINALIS is a remedy we have met before when we learned how Hahnemann came to discover the principles of Homeopathy. It is often very helpful for *traveler's diarrhea,* especially *after drinking contaminated water or fruit.* Typically there will be a lot of bloating and gas when CHINA is needed.

IPECACUANHA (IPECAC ROOT) is indicated when there is *severe cramping with persistent nausea and vomiting.* Years ago I treated a child with food poisoning with this remedy when the ARSENICUM given initially failed to completely eliminate the symptoms. A few doses of Homeopathic IPECAC did the trick. (This is not to be confused with Syrup of Ipecac, which used to be used to induce vomiting after ingestion of certain poisons.)

TRAUMA

First, let's cover some basic principles of Emergency Care.

In cases of acute trauma, the first things to remember are the ABCs: Airway, Breathing, and Circulation. A person can suffocate from an occluded airway faster than he or she can bleed to death. In cases of trauma or drowning, the first thing to do is to be sure the victim has a clear airway.

For choking, the Heimlich maneuver is the fastest way to clear the airway if a sharp slap to the back between the scapulas (the wing bones) doesn't clear the obstruction. It might be necessary to place your fingers in the victim's mouth or throat to clear any obstructions. (For a video demonstration on how to perform the Heimlich maneuver go to www.youtube.com/watch?v=tfDwIeBHo-M.)

Once the person is breathing, see if they are bleeding. Direct compression with a clean cloth (such as a shirt) directly over the wound is the first thing to do. If there is arterial bleeding, judicious application of a tourniquet is necessary to prevent acute exsanguination (bleeding out).

A tourniquet can be made from any kind of rod and a twisted piece of cloth. A stick, crowbar, or umbrella can be used to tighten the cloth placed around the limb. Be sure that the tourniquet is not so tight that it prevents all blood flow to the extremity. It is usually sufficient to reduce the blood flow to an ooze. Continued direct pressure can then be used to assist coagulation and stop bleeding.

Once the person is breathing and bleeding is stopped, he or she should be stabilized before being moved. *Never move a trauma victim without first securing his or her neck.* This is best left to the paramedics, who should have already been called.

After stabilization, remedies can be given. Vega Rozenberg taught me an important principle that he learned from the master homeopath George Vithoulkas. If you are ever in a situation and you have only one remedy, no matter what it is, give it. All homeopathic remedies are potentized and act on the Vital Force.

Though the available remedy might not be the simillimum, it will still have some effect in dire circumstances.

As you are stabilizing the person and arranging for transport to a hospital, the first remedy to give is ARNICA MONTANA.

An interesting fact about ARNICA is that it was selected for homeopathic proving after a homeopath observed the behavior of mountain goats: each time a goat fell, it immediately ate the Mountain Daisy plants known as ARNICA MONTANA. ARNICA provers developed bruising and pain similar to those resulting from trauma. Another curious fact about ARNICA is the mental state.

A person needing ARNICA after a traumatic event will often *deny that they are ill* and try to convince you they don't need to go to the hospital. I remember a patient I cared for in medical school who was in the Intensive Care Unit after suffering a heart attack and he kept insisting he was fine and kept trying to get out of bed. He eventually needed to be restrained but I now realize we could have spared the restraints if we had known to give him ARNICA.

Once the acute situation has passed, it is helpful to continue to give ARNICA for several days or weeks until there has been a full recovery.

CARBO VEGETABILIS is indicated in trauma cases where the person is *pale and has difficulty breathing.* Once again, be sure there is nothing obstructing the airway as the cause for breathing difficulty.

ACONITUM NAPELLUS is a remedy we discussed earlier for colds and in case of shock. In cases of acute trauma, ACONITE is very helpful for any kind of shock: physical, emotional or mental. [See 9/11 pg 59.]

HEAT EXHAUSTION AND HEAT STROKE

These are conditions commonly seen in the sunny southwestern U.S. Heatstroke is a severe form of heat exhaustion brought on by prolonged heat exposure. The body dissipates heat by sweating, and if this cooling mechanism is overwhelmed, heat stroke ensues.

Those most at risk for heatstroke include infants, elderly patients with chronic diseases who are on certain medications, outdoor workers, and athletes. The symptoms of heat exhaustion include nausea, vomiting, fatigue, weakness, headaches, muscle cramps, and dizziness.

Heatstroke is a life-threatening emergency where the body temperature exceeds 104°F. A leading cause of heatstroke is dehydration. Heatstroke can mimic the symptoms of a heart attack. Heatstroke symptoms can progress from heat exhaustion or they can come on suddenly without warning.

Symptoms of heatstroke include *high body temperature* and absence of sweating with hot, red, or flushed, dry skin. Victims also can have a rapid pulse, difficulty breathing, strange behavior, hallucinations, agitation, disorientation, seizures, or coma.

The first and most important thing to do for a victim of heatstroke is to cool the body. Remove the victim from heat by transferring them to an air-conditioned car or building. Remove their clothes and apply cool or tepid water to the skin. Place ice packs in the armpits and on both sides of the groin. You can also spray victims with cool water and fan them to promote cooling from evaporation. If they are conscious, give them cool liquids to drink that do not contain alcohol or caffeine.

Never attempt to give liquids to an unconscious person due to the risk of choking. As the cooling process continues, begin homeopathic remedies immediately.

The following are the remedies most often indicated for heatstroke: BELLADONNA is indicated when the victim is hot, irritable and has a bright red face. GLONOINUM, which is made from nitroglycerine, is indicated when the person complains of a headache that feels like the top of his or her head will explode; it is also indicated for people with explosive tempers or extreme irritability.

GRANATUM, made from pomegranate, is also an important remedy for heatstroke. This remedy is indicated when the entire body is hot, the skin is dry and there is a great thirst for water. They may also complain of nausea and abdominal cramps.

HEAD INJURY

HYPERICUM and NATRUM SULPHURICUM are two remedies for head trauma that should be given together. In most cases, the person will respond to either one, but in an emergency, give them both.

HYPERICUM and NATRUM SULPHURICUM are remedies especially for damage to areas rich in nerves. This includes the spine, the brain, the tips of the fingers, and the genitals. Along with RUTA and ARNICA, HYPERICUM is a remedy for *sciatica after trauma*. HYPERICUM alone is the remedy for damage to the peripheral nerves, but if there is damage to the spine and brain as well, give both HYPERICUM and NATRUM SULHURICUM.

Several years ago, I was making hospital rounds one morning and met a medical colleague in the corridor. He was obviously in pain as he hobbled along. I asked him what was wrong, and he told me that approximately three months earlier, while climbing Camelback Mountain, he fell on his left hip.

Since then, he had terrible pain in his sciatic nerve, with constant "pins and needles" sensations running down his leg. He was an avid cyclist but had not been able to ride his bike since the accident. He had had several epidural injections of steroids in his back, without relief.

His doctor told him that he would just have to "suffer through it" and prescribed narcotics. But the pain medications were so strong, he couldn't function very well, limping along and trying to care for his patients. I sent him a vial of HYPERICUM 200C and had him take one dose daily.

About a month later, I again saw my colleague at the hospital. He did a little dance for me and said that he was entirely pain-free after only ten doses. A properly chosen remedy can work wonders, even after an acute injury has had time to become chronic. However, in such cases, it might take several months of homeopathic treatment to restore the Vital Force, and hence the body, to complete health.

NATRUM SULPHURICUM is the remedy of choice for people with seizures after head injury. In chronic cases, it's the first remedy to try for people who have depression or emotional changes after head injury.

NATRUM SULPHURICUM is also a remedy to think of in cases of spinal meningitis, where the tissues that line the brain and the spinal chord are inflamed.

OPIUM is the remedy for coma after head injury. This is usually needed in cases where the person didn't get HYPERICUM or NATRUM SULPHURICUM quickly enough and has lapsed into a coma.

Note: In cases of head injury, the remedy needs to be repeated frequently. If the lower potency of 30C stops working, go up to 200C. Of course, this is not meant to be a substitute for professional care. But in cases where trauma occurs far from a hospital, properly given homeopathic remedies can save lives. Every outdoorsman should carry a homeopathic Emergency Kit and know how to use it. I am especially indebted to Vega Rozenberg who taught this information during a seminar at ESSH in August, 2009.

PUNCTURES and WOUNDS

LEDUM and APIS are companion remedies most frequently indicated when there has been a puncture of any kind including from insect bites, sharp objects or surgical needle biopsies. If the puncture site is *red, swollen and tender*, APIS is the correct remedy. When the wound is white or purple, use LEDUM.

VESPA is a helpful remedy in cases where there is *sharp, stinging pain* as in a scorpion bite.

CARBOLIC ACID is the remedy to give when there has been *an allergic response to a bee sting.*

HEART ATTACK

The first thing to do when you suspect someone is having a myocardial infarction (heart attack) is to get the person to a hospital. But while you're waiting for the ambulance, there are several remedies to give. The first is ACONITE, the remedy for shock. ACONITE is indicated when the person has feelings of extreme fatigue. You might need to repeat the ACONITE every few minutes and continue to do so even after they are in the hospital.

Vega Rozenberg tells the story of the song-and-dance man from the 1940s, Danny Kaye, who appreciated homeopathy and always carried remedies with him when he traveled. Mr. Kaye told about being on an airplane when the passenger seated next to him had a heart attack; he gave the man ACONITE.

The next remedy to give after ACONITE is CACTUS. CACTUS is indicated when the person complains of squeezing pain in the chest.

LATRODECTAS MACTANS, derived from the black widow spider, is required in cases where the chest pain is sharp and stabbing.

ARNICA MONTANA may also be indicated, especially if the person *denies they are sick* and refuses help.

SURGERY

Sometimes, despite the best efforts of a good homeopath, a client requires surgery. Surgery should rarely be the first choice of treatment, except in cases of acute trauma such as those resulting from motor vehicle accidents or gunshot wounds.

Even appendicitis and acute gall bladder attacks can be treated homeopathically if the homeopath can properly see the totality of symptoms and choose the right remedies.

There are several remedies that can make for a faster recovery and lessen the amount and duration of medications needed postoperatively. Homeopathy can also help to remove the toxic affects of general anesthesia.

ARNICA MONTANA – Surgery is essentially controlled trauma, and ARNICA is the *sine qua non* for trauma. I have my clients take one 30C dose under the tongue on their way to the hospital. This does not interfere with the usual advice to taking nothing by mouth after midnight, which aims to prevent vomiting by having the patient's stomach empty at the induction of anesthesia. After surgery, I have my clients take the remedy under the tongue every eight hours, usually for several weeks.

They can bring the remedies to the hospital and keep them in their shaving/make-up kits. I often write an order for the nurses such as this: "Patient may take their own homeopathic remedies from home."

In twenty-seven years of working in hospitals, I have never had a problem with my patients using their own remedies from home while in the hospital

STAPHYSAGRIA – This remedy does double duty: it not only helps prevent wound infections, but it also relieves the *painful urination* that occurs as a result of *bladder catheterization*. I often find that STAPHYSAGRIA allows me to avoid giving my clients "prophylactic" antibiotics that are routinely given during surgery. This remedy does not need to be given preoperatively but is also given every eight hours in the 30C potency, along with ARNICA.

RUTA is a mainstay for Orthopedic surgery, especially when the periosteum of the bones and the deep tissues of the muscles are involved. This is especially helpful after *total joint replacement*.

STRONTIUM CARBONICUM is a very good remedy for surgical shock after a prolonged operation with massive blood loss as is often seen in trauma cases requiring blood transfusion.

STRONTIUM CARBONCIUM is also used for the chronic effect of blood loss due to oozing. ACONITE would also be indicated for shock.

HAMAMELLIS is also helpful for postoperative bleeding. Several years ago there was a problem with a batch of suture sent to my hospital. This particular type of suture is designed to last for about six weeks and then dissolve. But as a result of one batch of defective suture, several of my surgical patients started to bleed prematurely from their incisions just three days post-op.

I happened to be at an ESSH seminar and Vega Rozenberg suggested I have the clients take HAMAMELLIS every 15 minutes. Within 3 doses, the bleeding stopped and I did not have to take any of them back to surgery. This is yet another example of the many useful Homeopathic "tricks of the trade" that I have learned over the years from Vega Rozenberg.

BISMUTH – This is a priceless remedy, as it often saves surgical patients from unnecessary pain, the discomfort of a nasogastric tube, and extra days in the hospital. *Ileus* is a common complication of abdominal surgery where the colon is slow to recover its normal function. Gas accumulates in the gut and causes severe pain with marked abdominal distention.

A few doses of BISMUTH 30C every thirty minutes work like a charm.

ARSENICUM ALBUM and GELSEMIUM SEMPERVIRENS are two remedies that are very helpful in cases where clients are slow to recover from the effects of general anesthesia.

ARSENICUM is indicated when the client complains of prolonged nausea or diarrhea.

GELSEMIUM is helpful in cases of lingering fatigue where the patient is slow to recover after surgery. Usually a dose of 30C daily for several days to a week post-op is enough to resolve the symptoms.

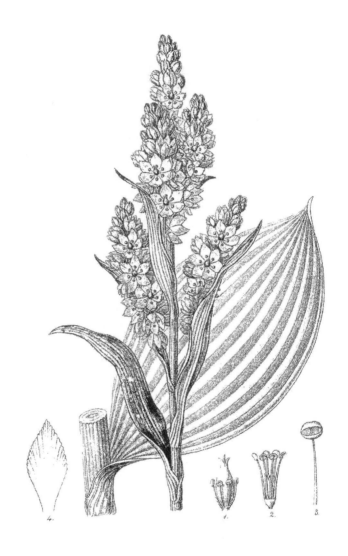

VERATRUM ALBUM

ACUTE REMEDIES FOR CHILDREN

One of the best books ever written about caring for children is *"Natural Baby, Healthy Child"* by Dr. Murray Clarke. Originally trained in Chinese medicine, Dr. Clarke is a Naturopathic Physician as well as a one of the best homeopaths working in the world today. He has more than twenty-five years of experience treating children in Los Angeles. His book is a brilliant guide for parents who are looking for successful alternatives to conventional allopathic treatment for their children.

You can purchase the book online at Amazon. The chapter on vaccination alone is worth 100 times the cost of the book and a must read for any parent looking for excellent, science based information on this crucial topic.

Teething is a common problem for babies, and often a source of frustration and anguish for parents. Fortunately, Homeopathy is a safe and very effective way to relieve babies' suffering and stop the crying.

The first remedy to think of for crying babies with *teething pain and drooling* is CHAMOMILLA VULGARIS. These babies are very cross, and their pain seems intolerable. They *insist on being held*, usually high up on the shoulder, and like to be carried around fast. Sometimes one dose of a 30C is enough to relieve the pain. Watch carefully and repeat the dose as needed.

CHAMOMILLA is also the first remedy to try for colic, especially when the baby is very fussy, wants to be held all the time, and climbs up the mother's shoulder, pressing the belly into the shoulder. Instead of driving your child around the neighborhood at midnight or putting her on top of a dryer while it's running, try a dose of CHAMOMILLA and be grateful for the miracle of a good night's sleep for the entire household.

CHAMOMILLA is also very helpful for earaches brought on

by exposure to wind. The classic symptom that is a hallmark of CHAMOMILLA is one red cheek and one pale cheek.

Nothing brings more pain to children and more anguish to parents than ear infections (Otitis media). In Dr. Clarke's book *"Natural Baby, Healthy Child,"* he discusses many ways parents can help prevent such infections.

There are several remedies that no home with small children should be without. FERRUM PHOSPHORICUM, GELSEMIUM, and CHAMOMILLA are commonly indicated remedies for cases of Otitis media. (See above.)

Other remedies that are often indicated depending on the symptom presentation include the following:

BELLADONNA. This remedy is often indicated for children who have had multiple ear infections. BELLADONNA is the remedy to choose when there is *sudden onset of ear pain*, usually *starting in the right ear*, often accompanied by a very *high fever and a flushed face.* Start with a 30C and repeat the remedy every hour until the fever comes down. BELLADONNA is usually a short-acting remedy indicated for conditions that come on quickly and leave quickly.

PULSATILLA is a wonderful remedy especially for children with ear infections associated with chickenpox. In fact, giving PULSATILLA at the first sign of chickenpox will often prevent an ear infection. Children needing PULSATILLA are often clingy and very moody. They feel better being in the open air and tend to be chilly and thirstless. They are also very whiny and can cry for long periods of time.

MERCURIUS SOLUBULIS HAHNEMANN (MERCURY) (Yes, it's made from what was used in old thermometers.) This is the remedy to think of when children have swollen tonsils with enlarged lymph glands in the neck and foul-smelling breath. The children often drool in their sleep and awaken with puddles on their pillows.

SILICA, made from flint, is another very useful remedy for children. Children needing SILICA have a tendency to be easily exhausted, especially after vaccinations. It's a common remedy for children with recurring ear infections who are slow in mental or physical development.

The hallmark of SILICA is a pathological *fear of needles.* Oftentimes the children have unhealthy skin and brittle nails with white spots on them. Silica is a classic remedy to extrude foreign objects such as splinters.

A client of mine once had small pieces of glass embedded in her face after going through the windshield in a car accident. You could feel the glass particles just under the surface of the skin. SILICA caused the glass particles to come out on her pillow at night. All of the glass was removed within about a year and she was able to stop taking the Silica.

I can't conclude this brief summary of remedies for children without saying something about vaccinations. When you understand the true nature of disease, you see why vaccinations are so problematic. A multitude of "morbific agents inimical to life" are actually injected into your child simultaneously. Remember that everything in Nature has both a physical and a spiritual component.

When you vaccinate your child, you are injecting them with the spirit of something that causes death and disease.

The most comprehensive treatment on this subject can be found in *"Natural Baby, Healthy Child"* by Dr. Murray Clarke. In the chapter on vaccination, Dr. Clarke makes a very valid point that I had never considered. When in your child's life is he or she ever going to be in a situation where they would *simultaneously* be exposed to Diphtheria, Pertussis, Tetanus, Hepatitis B, Hemophilus Influenza, Polio, Mumps, Measles, German Measles, and Chickenpox?

Following what the American Academy of Pediatrics recommends, your child will have received 32 vaccinations by the age of two years and a total of 43 by age five.

Children nowadays receive many more vaccines than they

did even a generation ago. I am convinced that, along with our polluted environment and pesticide-laden food, massive vaccination is one of the contributing factors to the epidemic we are now seeing of children with Autism Spectrum Disorders, Attention Deficit Disorder, and Attention Deficit Hyperactivity Disorder.

I highly recommend that you read Dr. Clarke's book, and especially the thoughtful and very thorough chapter on vaccination. Reading this book will help you to make an informed decision about vaccinations and to be able to discuss the subject intelligently with your child's pediatrician.

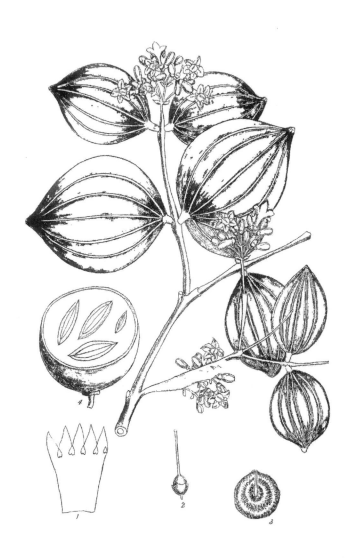

NUX VOMICA

ACUTE REMEDIES FOR WOMEN

As a gynecologist caring for women for more than twenty-seven years, I have had many occasions to use Homeopathy for acute problems in addition to completely removing long-standing diseases.

Homeopathy works miracles for couples with *unexplained infertility*. By definition, this is a condition where there are no anatomical or hormonal reasons why a couple is not conceiving a child. The woman is producing eggs, and there are no blockages in her Fallopian tubes that carry the sperm to the egg. The man has a normal semen analysis with an adequate number of normally shaped, motile sperm.

Taking the woman's case and putting her on a remedy often results in conception. On rare occasions, the husband will also need homeopathic treatment as well.

One of the most dramatic cases I treated was that of Lori and Steve. They had been married for three years and had been trying to get pregnant for the past two years. The extensive infertility evaluation they had endured was completely normal. In desperation they were considering in vitro fertilization.

Lori was reluctant to take hormones because she had not reacted well in the past to oral contraceptives. They were also very concerned about the expense which was not covered by their insurance plan.

They had a friend with the same condition who had a child after taking a remedy I had recommended for her, so Lori and Steve were ready to try Homeopathy. Lori happened to have her case taken during the middle of her menstrual cycle when she was ovulating. I recommended a remedy for her, which she took that day; within four weeks, she called to report a positive pregnancy test. Lori continued the remedy throughout her pregnancy, and nine months later she and Steve became proud and happy parents of a nine-pound baby boy without expensive drug treatments.

Although conception doesn't always happen this quickly, Homeopathy is the treatment of choice for couples with *unexplained infertility.*

The following is a brief overview of some of the most common remedies used for women with various conditions.

Mastitis is a common condition in nursing mothers characterized by a hot, swollen and inflamed area of the breast, often around the nipple. It is extremely painful, and conventional medicine treats it with antibiotics. Oftentimes, mothers are encouraged to stop nursing so the baby doesn't get the antibiotics through the milk.

Sometimes drugs are given to dry up the mother's milk and the baby is then deprived of its best source of nutrition. PHYTOLACCA 30C every one to two hours is a miracle remedy for nursing mothers. The redness and swelling quickly subside, and there is no need to stop nursing, because the remedy has no harmful effect on the baby.

PHYTOLACCA also can be used to treat chronic mastitis. A few years ago, one of my clients, Marianne, developed a severe case of mastitis of the left breast. When she came to see me, she had a painful, tennis-ball-size red area on her left breast. It was so tender and swollen that she couldn't bear to have anything touch her skin, much less wear a bra.

She had a fever of 100.9°F and a blood-tinged discharge from the nipple. The interesting thing about Marianne's case was that she had developed a case of mastitis in the exact same place on the same breast while she was nursing her son more than thirty-five years ago. Of course, at that time she was given antibiotics and told to stop nursing.

Because Marianne has had good homeopathic treatment since 2005, this condition is the result of the constitutional remedy annihilating a disease that had been suppressed for thirty-five years. This is called *"return of old symptoms."*

When Marianne's mastitis returned, I gave her four hourly doses of PHYTOLACCA 30C, the remedy she needed thirty-five years ago. Her temperature dropped to 99.9°F with minor improvement in her level of pain. I increased her constitutional remedy, MAGNESIUM CARBONICUM, to LM34 daily and had her go up to PHYTOLACCA 200C every two hours through the night.

The following day, she had no fever and felt considerably better, with less tenderness and considerably less redness.

She continued PHYTOLACCA 200C every hour and I had her order the next higher potency of PHYTOLACCA, 1M (1,000C), just in case it was needed. Because inflammatory breast cancer can present this way, I sent her for a breast MRI, which was suspicious for ductal carcinoma in situ, an early form of breast cancer.

We increased the remedy to PHYTOLACCA 1M daily, and she got three opinions regarding the diagnosis. It was agreed that a biopsy was warranted, and I concurred. The biopsy revealed a benign *intraductal papilloma*, a simple polyp.

She continued PHYTOLACCA 1M daily, the abscess slowly resolved, and the nipple discharge became clear yellow. After four months, all the breast symptoms resolved, and the PHYTOLACCA was stopped.

Marianne's case is a good example of how Homeopathy can be used to restore a person to health even after something has been suppressed for decades. In addition, Marianne's underlying chronic conditions, for which she started Homeopathy, improved markedly. She continues to take her constitutional remedy, and we continue to see steady improvement in her overall health.

One of the most debilitating conditions I see in my clinic is *Premenstrual Syndrome.* A client's husband often brings his wife in, complaining that he doesn't know what happened to the woman he married. She's *cranky and irritable,* especially prior to her menses. Not only does she have no sexual desire—she can't bear to be touched.

This is very common, especially for women who have taken birth control pills for years and also have had children. In evaluating these women homeopathically, they often tell me that they crave chocolate and sour foods, love dancing, and get excited during thunderstorms.

They will often have a brown "mask of pregnancy" over their cheeks. The remedy indicated here is SEPIA, made from the ink of the cuttlefish, a close relative of the squid. Once they start taking this remedy, their disposition gradually improves, and their sexual desire returns. There are many grateful husbands out there thanks to the action of SEPIA.

One of my favorite homeopathic stories is about how Hahnemann came to discover the healing powers of Sepia. Hahnemann had a client under his care for several chronic conditions. He had tried several remedies to help him without relief. He decided to make a home visit to see the man in his own environment hoping to find a clue to the remedy needed. Visiting the man at home, Hahnemann discovered him painting, using ink made from the cuttlefish. As Hahnemann watched the man repeatedly lick the brush after dipping it into the ink, it was clear to him that the man was doing a proving on himself of Sepia. By preparing a homeopathic remedy from the cuttlefish ink and giving it to the man in potentized form, Hahnemann was able to permanently relieve his symptoms. We owe our knowledge of this very important remedy, especially for women, to Hahnemann's persistent and keen powers of observation.

Nothing is more distressing (or common) for women than *urinary tract infections.* As previously discussed, these often appear after intercourse and after catheterization for surgical procedures.

The most common complaint of women with urinary tract infections (UTIs) is frequency and urgency of urination; often there is an intense desire to void, but very little liquid is passed. Sometimes there is blood in the urine, or it may have a foul odor to it. There are several remedies that work for UTIs depending on the totality of symptoms.

STAPHYSAGRIA is probably the most common remedy given for UTI symptoms. The most common indication for this remedy is "honeymoon cystitis." It is also the remedy for women with urinary symptoms after sexual assault or sexual abuse. And it's the most common remedy used in women who develop symptoms after bladder catheterization for childbirth or surgical procedures.

STAPHYSAGRIA is also indicated for chronic conditions associated with suppressed anger or after severe humiliation or punishment. It is helpful to prevent wound infections in surgical patients.

CANTHARIS, a remedy made from "Spanish fly," is a remedy for bladder infections following repeated sexual relations. The pain is described as cutting and is so severe that sometimes women scream with pain that usually occurs at the end of urination; there is an intense desire to void constantly.

One of the consequences of *untreated urinary tract infections* can be a kidney infection (pyelonephritis). While most urinary tract infections are confined to the bladder, if the infection is not properly treated it can extend up the ureters into the kidneys. This is usually associated with flank tenderness and fever.

The classic sign of *pyelonephritis* is acute pain when the flank is palpated. This is a serious infection and should be treated by a professional homeopath. Improperly treated kidney infections can lead to lasting kidney disease. In cases of severe infection with fever, flank pain, and a large amount of pus in the urine, PYROGENIUM is often indicated. *Pyelonephritis* can also result from *obstruction* of the flow of urine by *kidney stones* either in the kidneys or in the ureters.

The first remedy to consider for kidney stones is BERBERIS VULGARIS. This remedy is indicated when there is severe pain from a kidney stone, usually characterized by extreme spastic pain.

It has been said that only childbirth is more painful than passing a kidney stone. Start with a 30C every thirty minutes. If there is minimal response after three or four doses, go up to a 200C every one to two hours. This will usually help the client to pass the stone.

BERBERIS can also be used for gallstone colic associated

with jaundice and pain shooting up into the left shoulder. Usually the pains radiate out from one point, and the client can usually point to a specific place where the pain starts.

In addition to those remedies listed above in the section on surgery, one of the most helpful yet underused remedies for women undergoing gynecological surgery is BELLIS PERENNIS.

Made from a daisy, it is often referred to as the "ARNICA of the pelvis." BELLIS PERENNIS is very helpful for women with persistent abdominal pain after pelvic surgery. I have also used it successfully, together with APIS, for pelvic thrombophlebitis, a condition where blood clots form in the pelvic veins, usually after surgery or pelvic inflammatory disease.

Entire books have been written on the uses of homeopathic remedies in assisting women through *pregnancy and in childbirth* [See REFRENCES]. In an ideal world, women would deliver their babies at home, attended by loving people well versed in how to use Homeopathy during labor and delivery.

The information provided here is not meant to be a substitute for professional care with a physician or midwife. My hope is that more childbirth attendants will discover and use Homeopathy for the benefit of their clients.

The following is a brief overview of some of the remedies that are particularly helpful in childbirth.

CIMICIFUGA (made from black cohosh) is very helpful for women with morning sickness. It has been used to ensure living births for women who have had repeated stillbirths. Given before term, it is thought to make labor easier. CIMICIFUGA is the remedy to use when labor slows and the mother is very emotional.

CAULOPHYLLUM (made from blue cohosh) is a miraculous remedy for pregnant women and laboring mothers. It is quite helpful in preventing miscarriage, especially for women with recurrent miscarriages. I once attended a laboring mother whose baby was Occiput Posterior, meaning that the baby's head was banging against her sacrum. As she approached the transitional stage of labor, her contractions became weaker.

After one dose of CAULOPHYLLUM 30C, the baby turned, and the mother's severe back pain immediately stopped. A healthy baby boy was born within twenty minutes.

ACONITE is a Godsend during labor and delivery, as it helps to calm the anxiety mothers often feel while in labor. It is the most important remedy for premature labor and is also very effective for the baby if there are any breathing difficulties after birth. Transient tachypnea of the newborn is a condition where the baby's breathing is very rapid and shallow and comes primarily from the chest.

A few doses of ACONITE 30C usually can restore a baby's breathing to a normal pattern, which is more rapid than ours and comes from deep in the belly. If the baby is pale and the breathing labored, CARBO VEGETABILIS is also indicated.

CALENDULA tincture applied directly to any tears or episiotomy of the perineum heals the lacerations like glue. This is the only time we use a MOTHER TINCTURE directly on the skin, rather than a potentized remedy.

CALENDULA, the primary remedy for bleeding, is also helpful in cases where oozing of blood continues. However, in cases of deep lacerations through the vagina, perineum and even in to the rectum, CALENDULA tincture is NOT a substitute for proper surgical repair.

BELLADONNA is a life-saving remedy for sudden onset of postpartum hemorrhage where the blood is hot and bright red, as opposed to dark and clotted. This is also the first remedy to use if there is bleeding from a retained placenta. If the bleeding is severe, the 200C potency should be used and repeated very frequently until the bleeding stops and the placenta is expelled.

CHINA OFFICINALIS is also a remedy used for post partum bleeding that is prolonged and accompanied by weakness and anemia. It is the first remedy to consider for a woman with chronic fatigue ever since childbirth, especially if she required a blood transfusion due to hemorrhage.

CANTHARIS is indicated in cases of retained placenta with urinary obstruction and painful urination. Women needing CANTHARIS complain of burning pain and a constant urge to urinate. CANTHARIS is also indicated for *nymphomania after* childbirth, where sexual desire is greatly increased.

This is a quite distressing symptom for a woman who has just had a baby and needs pelvic rest. Usually one or two doses of CANTHARIS reduces the sexual drive to a normal level.

CARBO VEGETABILIS is indicated for retained placenta where the mother is pale and suffers from exhaustion after prolonged labor. If CARBO VEG doesn't relieve the fatigue, try GELSEMIUM.

CAULOPHYLLUM is also helpful in cases of retained placenta due to weak uterine contractions. One or two doses will usually cause the uterus to expel the placenta.

GELSEMIUM is especially helpful for women who become weak and very emotional during labor. The Repertory calls this symptom *"hysteria of pregnancy"*, and though the term is not very flattering, it is a not uncommon occurrence, especially in first births that tend to take considerable time.

GELSEMIUM 30C repeated as needed is very helpful in such cases. If the laboring mother does not respond to GELSEMIUM, IGNATIA is also very helpful for extreme emotions while in labor or after delivery.

CHAMOMILLA is also very helpful during childbirth when the mother suffers from "touchiness" and irritability and is hot and thirsty. Often just a few doses of 30C will help.

GOSSYPIUM HERBACEUM is a rarely employed remedy,

but it has a very specific use in childbirth. It is indicated when, after the child is born, the cervix clamps down tightly and completely closes. GOSSYPIUM (one or two doses) opens the internal cervical opening, and allows the placenta to be released.

IPECAC, KALI CARBONICUM, or NUX VOMICA can be used in cases of retained placenta accompanied by the hallmark symptoms of each remedy. The hallmark symptom of IPECAC is abdominal cramping, nausea and vomiting. KALI CARBONICUM is indicated in cases of retained placenta with back pain and sweating.

NUX VOMICA is indicated in cases of retained placenta with severe heartburn or stomach ache.

SEPIA is probably the most important remedy for various ailments following childbirth, and no homeopath caring for women can dare be without it. SEPIA is indicated for women who have *never felt well since childbirth*. I have successfully used this remedy for many women who years after childbirth continued to be plagued with *fatigue, irritability, and low sex drive.*

SEPIA has a very particular characteristic in that a woman needing it will complain of *aversion to the touch of her husband.* For women who have needed this remedy for years, SEPIA is often required for many months to several years to fully restore the woman to a normal state of sexual desire.

I cringe when I think of how many marriages have been destroyed over the years because women didn't get SEPIA when needed.

There are many other more chronic conditions that affect women, such as Endometriosis, Polycystic Ovarian Syndrome, and *severe vasomotor symptoms* related to the menopause. In these chronic cases, the help of a professional homeopath is needed.

I am often asked, "What's the one remedy I can take for my menopausal symptoms?" We know that Homeopathy doesn't work that way. Homeopathy works on the spirit, on the Vital Force. Therefore, each woman will need a different remedy based on her own totality of symptoms. It is only after thoroughly evaluating an entire case that a proper remedy can be chosen and properly administered following well-established principles.

CONCLUSION

Homeopathy is a powerful, subtle and deep acting system of healing. When used according to the principles elucidated by Samuel Hahnemann, M. D. it can be used to restore the very ill to a state of health, facilitate the delivery of healthy babies and ease the suffering of the dying.

Its principles are simple enough that with study and practice, you can learn to use homeopathic remedies for such common ailments as colds and flus. Understanding how the Spiritual Vital Force is affected when you become ill allows you to choose the proper remedy and restore your health without pharmaceutical drugs.

In cases of chronic illness, there is no substitute for a consultation with a professional homeopath experienced in taking care of the seriously ill.

I hope this introduction to the wonders of Homeopathy inspires you to further study and experience for yourself this miraculous blessing from Our Creator.

Kathleen K. Fry, MD, CTHHom.
April, 2013
Boulder, Colorado

REFERENCES

Boericke, William. *Materia Medica with Repertory, 9th Edition*. Boericke & Tafel, Inc. Santa Rosa, CA. (1927).

Clarke, John Henry. *Dictionary of Practical Materia Medica. Vol I-III. 3rd Edition*. Homeopathic Book Service, Sittingbourne, Kent, U.K. (1991).

Clarke, Murray. *Natural Baby, Healthy Child*. Authority Publishing, Gold River, CA. (2010).

Coulter, Harris. *Divided Legacy: A History of the Schism in Medical Thought*. North Atlantic Books, Berkeley, CA. (1994).

Hahnemann, Samuel. *Organon of Medicine, 6th Edition*, translated by William Boericke, Jain Publishers, New Delhi. (2001).

Hamilton, Edward. *The Flora Homoeopathica: or, Illustrations and Descriptions of the Medicinal Plants Used as Homoeopathic Remedies*, two volumes. H. Bailliere, London. (1852 and 1853).

Handley, Rima. *A Homeopathic Love Story: The Story of Samuel and Melanie Hahnemann*. North Atlantic Books. Homeopathic Educational Services, Berkeley, CA. (1990).

Idarius, Betty. *The Homeopathic Childbirth Manual: A Practical Guide for Labor, Birth and the Immediate Postpartum Period*. Idarius Press, Ukiah, CA. (1996).

Kent, James Tyler. *Lectures on Homeopathic Philosophy*. North Atlantic Books. Homeopathic Educational Services, Berkeley, CA. (1979).

Murphy, Robin. *Nature's Materia Medica, 3rd Edition*. Narayana Publishers, Toronto, Canada. (2006).

Sherr, Jeremy. Proving of Androctonos. Dynamis School for Advanced Homeopathic Studies. www.dynamis.edu.

Vithoulkas, George. *Homeopathy: Medicine of the New Man*. Simon & Schuster, New York. (1979).

RESOURCES

Homeopathic Pharmacies:

American Medical College of
Homeopathy
1951 West Camelback Rd. # 300
Phoenix, AZ 85015
(602) 347-7950

Arrowroot Standard Direct
Ltd.
83 East Lancaster Ave,
Paoli, PA 19301
(800) 234-8879
customerservice@arrowroot.com

Boericke and Tafel Inc.
2381 Circadian Way
Santa Rosa, CA 95407
(707) 571-8202
(707) 571-8237 fax

Boiron-Bornemann Inc.
Box 449
6 Campus Ave. Building A
Newton Square, PA 19073
(800) BLU-TUBE

Boiron-Bornemann Inc.
98c W. Cochran St.
Simi Valley, CA 93065
(800) 258-8823

Dolisos America Inc.
3014 Rigel Avenue
Las Vegas, NV 89102
(800) 365-4767

Hahnemann Laboratories,
Inc.1940 4th Street
San Rafael, CA 94901
(888) 427-6422
(415) 451-6978
www.hahnemannlabs.com

Natural Health Supply
6410 Avenida Christina
Santa Fe, NM 87507
(505) 474-9175
(888) 689 1608
(505) 473-0336 fax

Santa Monica Homeopathic
Pharmacy
629 Broadway
Santa Monica, CA 90401
(310) 395-1131
(310) 395-7861 fax
info@smhomopathic.com

Standard Homeopathic
Company
P.O. Box 61067
204-210 W. 131st St
Los Angeles, CA 90061
(800) 624-9659 Washington

Washington Homeopathic
Products Inc.
4915 Del Ray Avenue
Bethesda, MD 20814
(800) 336-1695
(301) 656-1847

Emergency Kit:
Hahnemann Labs Expanded Home Kit
www.hahnemannlabs.com - (888) 427 6642

GLOSSARY OF TERMS

Vital Force: According to Dr. Samuel Hahnemann, it is the "spirit-like dynamis" that controls all functions of any living creature, "with unbounded sway."

Homeopathy: A scientific and artful system of healing based on understanding and manipulating the spiritual Vital Force in order to annihilate "dis-ease" and restore health.

Proving: The process of determining the inherent, dynamic healing properties of a substance by observing its effects on healthy volunteers in a carefully supervised and thoroughly documented manner.

Materia Medica: The compilation of results of every proving ever conducted since Samuel Hahnemann, the Father of Homeopathy, undertook the first proving in the late 18th century.

Organon of Medicine: Samuel Hahnemann's "magnum opus" in which he elucidates the principles and methods of the healing art he named Homeopathy.

Mother Tincture: The original mixture of a substance with water or alcohol from which a homeopathic remedy is made by serial dilutions.

Simillimum: The one remedy which most closely corresponds to the totality of symptoms revealed by a thorough evaluation of the state of the subject's vital force.

Potency: The strength of a homeopathic remedy. As the number of dilutions of the Mother Tincture of a substance increases, the stronger the potency of the remedy.

ACKNOWLEDGEMENTS

It has been my privilege to share my passion for Homeopathy with you. Every day I marvel at its power. I thank God who gave us this beautiful healing art through the life and work of Dr. Samuel Hahnemann. I am grateful for all the homeopaths and teachers throughout the ages who have kept this knowledge alive so that many more may follow this path of true healing.

As an obstetrician by training, the analogy of labor and delivery of a child and the writing and publishing of a book is an apt one. This "baby" has had many doulas in its birthing and I am grateful to each of them for the help they gave me through this long labor.

First is my sister, Betsy Kolt Pausch for her emotional support, and who with her co-designer Roz Migdal, created a beautiful cover.

Greg Williams was invaluable in his role as my first editor and I wish him the most joyful of retirements.

Deborah Ledford, my faithful editor, kept me on track and skillfully "midwifed" this book in all its iterations.

I am so grateful to Lori Durfee, my long-term assistant who managed my office for more than sixteen years. Her capable attention to the daily details gave me the freedom to focus my attention on caring for my patients.

And last, but never least, this book could never have been written without my patients who give me the privilege of their trust and continue to inspire me with their commitment to their own healing.

23964424R00061

Made in the USA
San Bernardino, CA
07 September 2015